First published in Great Britain in 2014 by Unkant Publishers
2 Pascoe Road, London SE13 5JB

Designed by Keith Fisher and Andy Wilson
Cover illustration by Louise Challice
Author photograph by Gini Simpson
Mad Pride logo by Penny Shaughnessy
Editorial Assistance by Ted Curtis

British Library Cataloguing-in-Publication Data
A CIP catalogue record for this book is available from the British Library
A Paperback Original

ISBN 978-0-9926509-0-2
1 3 5 7 9 10 8 6 4 2

Set in Unkant Jensen
www.unkant.com

Splitting in Two

Mad Pride and Punk Rock Oblivion

Robert Dellar

Unkant Publishers
London

Contents

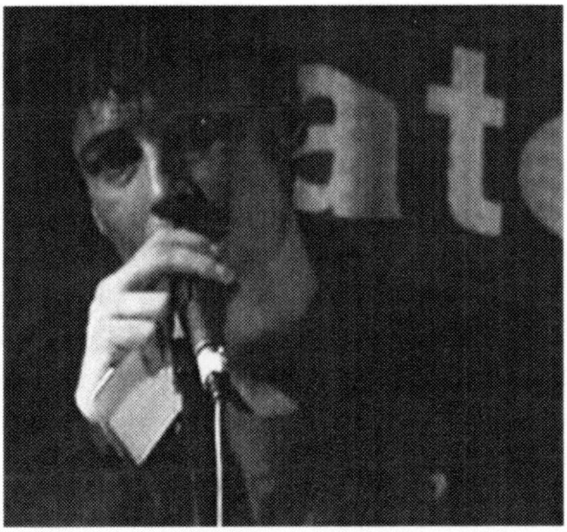

Robert Dellar

Robert Dellar has worked for various mental health charities since 1987, helping to pioneer advocacy and survivor-led projects. Beginning with the punk fanzine *Breach of the Peace,* he has published underground magazines prolifically since 1980, most recently *Southwark Mental Health News.* He is editor of *Gobbing, Pogoing and Gratuitous Bad Language: An Anthology of Punk Short Stories* (1996), co-author of the novel *Seaton Point* (1998), co-editor of *Mad Pride: A Celebration of Mad Culture* (2000), and has featured in numerous anthologies. Setting up Mad Pride with three friends in 1999 allowed him to fuse his long-term preoccupations with madness, leftist political provocation and outsider rock 'n' roll. He lives in South London with his partner Shirley. *Splitting in Two* is the first book entirely of his own writing.

Note From the Publishers

We are amazed at the life and times of Robert Dellar, and believe his work deserves the widest consideration. However, given the fact that he has obviously imbibed deep and long at the fountains of freedom and invention provided by London Psychogeography we would like to say that we love what he says for its general truth, but do not believe anyone should take literally the details of his account of any particular event, real or imagined.

This is literature not journalism.

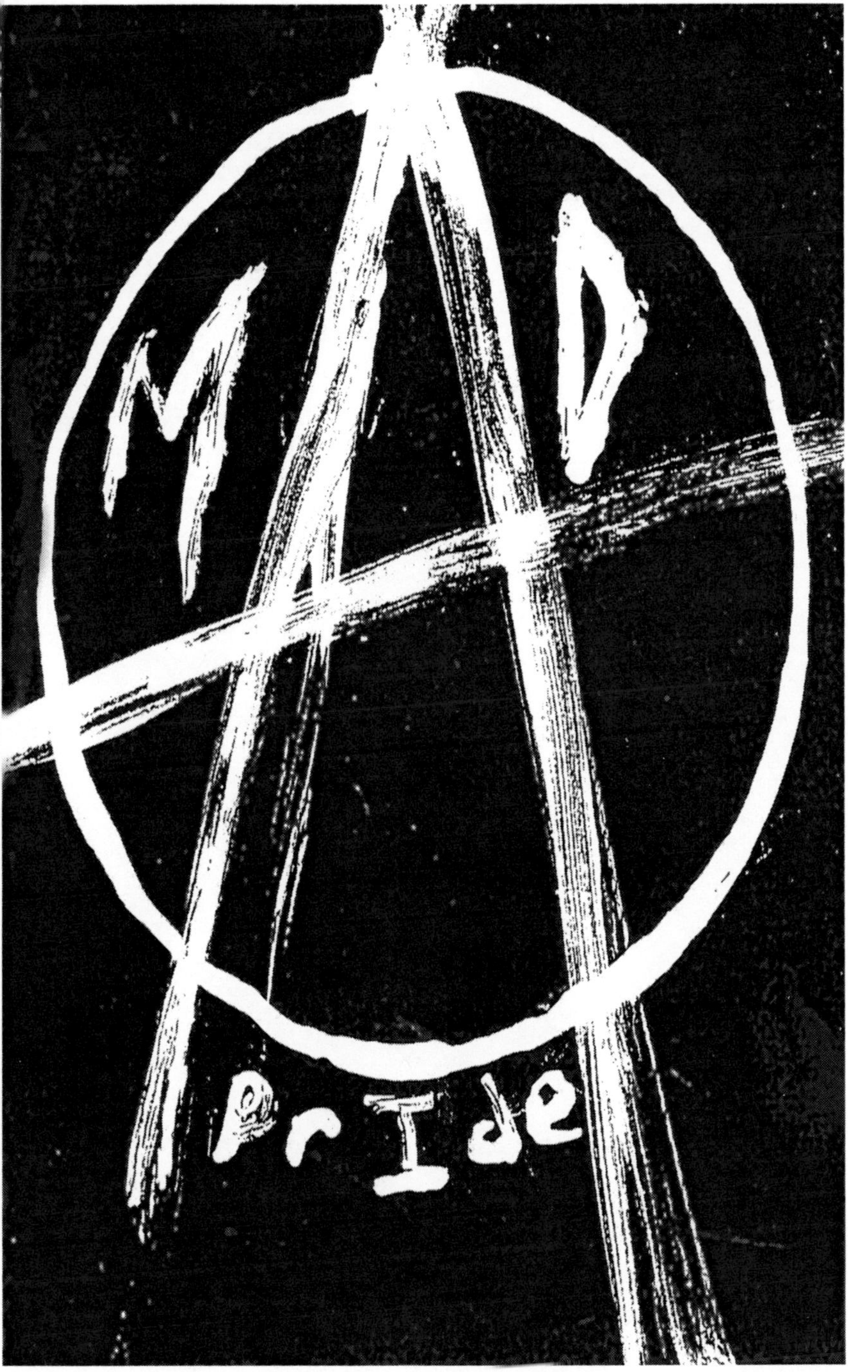
MAD
prIde

Problem Child

I arrived at work at one o'clock in the afternoon. It was January 2003 and I was coordinator of the Southwark branch of Mind, a nationwide mental health charity with a network of local and barely-related affiliated groups. Southwark is a borough in South East London which includes Peckham, Camberwell, Bermondsey and Rotherhithe. Compared to other Mind groups, we were almost unique in terms of being entirely managed and staffed by people with mental health problems, and successful. The office in Camberwell was hard to get to from Hackney, and the progressive deterioration of the public transport system had added hours to my journey to and from Southwark since I'd first started helping to set up the charity in 1998. But I got on with it, and as was often the case, I had a bad hangover from the day before and I'd been topping myself up on the way in.

By now I'd already handed in my notice. Fifteen years at the cutting edge of mental health services takes its toll, and depression and heavy drinking had crept up on me. I wanted space to sort myself out, and hoped to tidy up some of the loose ends at Southwark Mind before I left. Some chance.

Stumbling into the office, I was informed by our admin officer Teresa Priest and volunteer Robert Radford that our chair, Lynne Clayton, had commanded that I was not allowed to be at work because I was 'too ill'. She was right, though at the time it was a case of the pot calling the kettle black: Lynne was as high as a kite. *"I'll phone the office in an hour"* she told me over the blower. *"Time enough for you to have a cup of tea. If you're still there in an hour, I'll come and physically escort you off the premises."*

Lynne wasn't joking. Although small and apparently frail, she had a black belt in karate. You messed about with her at your peril, and rumour had it that her several hospital admissions had been made easier for her by her skill in the martial arts.

Feeling a bit rejected, I went down the pub. I tried to help keep Southwark Mind ticking from the pleasant afternoon environment of Monaghan's bar, using my walkie-talkie, and I completed a Disability Living Allowance (DLA) form for my friend, Ted Curtis, over a few beers. DLA forms are notoriously painstaking to complete. They're fifty pages long and require almost novel-length accounts of woe in exchange for the substantial amounts of money due to the recipient if anyone can be bothered to complete them. On these forms, you have to pretend that you don't know your arse from your elbow. It's been the difference between poverty and survival for tens of thousands of people. You have to wallow in your incapacity in writing at great length and, for my sins, I have acquired the knack of filling in these miserable things, benefiting a great many people. I have cost the decent, honest taxpayer a fortune.

Prior to this it had been a difficult few months, full of tragedy and high stress. After various people committing suicide, people around me being ill all the time and numerous demanding situations both domestically and at work, all of it was compounded by the death of my friend and Mad Pride colleague Pete Shaughnessy, who threw himself under a train at Battersea on December 15th 2002. I was informed of the event by mental health activist Cath Collins the following day, my 38th birthday. Pete's death knocked me sideways and convinced me after several months of thinking about it that it was time for me to blow out my job. Life seemed too short to spend all of it being a wage slave, especially since I realised that I was no longer the most competent person for the post.

Somebody had to pay. To cheer myself up, back in Hackney I walked up to B&Qs in Lea Bridge Road to buy a power drill. Returning home along the cycle path which doubled as a footpath towards Upper Clapton, a cyclist approached shouting *"get out of the fucking way you stupid cunt!"* One little nudge was all it took. Straight into the path of an oncoming lorry. Splat! It wasn't my fault, it was just one of those things. I used my walkie-talkie to call emergency services, but it was too late: the cyclist was dead. It's bad when that happens.

Things like this made me want to reflect on how it was that I had arrived at this situation. Self-indulgence is a vice I sometimes try to avoid, but who knows, I thought, something could come out of it that might help chart part of the rise of the mental health service user movement, in which I've been far from a disinterested observer.

Splitting in Two is a catchy title, and also one of the best songs by one of my favourite bands, Alternative TV, run by Mark Perry, who has unwittingly been a major influence on me. For a start, the layout of *Southwark Mind Newsletter,* which I edited over consecutive, uninterrupted months for 61 issues prior to my resignation, was ripped off wholesale from Mark's fanzine *Sniffin' Glue* which he edited during 1976 and 1977. 'Splitting in Two' was also the final song performed, by ATV, at the tribute concert for Pete Shaughnessy, held by Mad Pride at the Garage, North London, on summer solstice night 2003. Music has always been a major preoccupation of mine and has affected my approach to work and life generally in many ways. I don't know how anyone manages without it.

More pretentiously, *Splitting in Two* can refer to the dialectical model of philosophical and political analysis first elucidated by Hegel and then developed by Marx. Loosely, dialectics consists of separating elements of received ideas, situations and facts into opposing and contradictory parts, contrasting them, and allowing the ensuing contradictions to stimulate higher, better approaches and methods of thought. This is how human progress is made. As human beings, we are unable to advance from what faces us without such a process. Our social being consists to begin with only of what we encounter and what we absorb, and advancement is possible only through deliberately applied reason, not magic or genius. Dialectical analysis allows political and scientific development. You won't find much dialectics in here, but hopefully it may feed into a dialectical process somewhere along the line. Ben Watson is very hot on the subject: check out his book *Art, Class and Cleavage.*[1]

---

1. Ben Watson, *Art, Class and Cleavage: Quantalumcunque Concerning Materialist Esthetics,* London, Quartet, 1998.

Splitting in Two also reminds me of R.D. Laing's seminal mental health book *The Divided Self*, which attempted to make some forms of madness comprehensible within a materialist framework, through debunking the myth that what is labelled 'schizophrenia' can be reduced to 'split personality'. Laing too has been a great inspiration for me, more because of his numerous and committed caring initiatives than his theories, which are at times unempirical. I've also shared with him an often dangerous lifestyle, and a propensity to burn myself out. Overall, *Splitting in Two* is a phrase rooted firmly within the punk tradition, and it accurately describes my state of mind and that of most of my friends, much of the time.

As with any undertaking involving memory, what follows is selective and at times inaccurate. I've censored my writing out of a wish not to upset anyone who wasn't asking for it, to avoid dwelling on things which are too awkward, and to protect myself from consequences. Some names have been altered to protect confidentiality. I don't consider my experiences to be any more important or interesting than anyone else's, though recalling some provides a context for various observations, which may or may not be taken with a pinch of salt.

I was born in 1964 into a not well off and, in most respects, stereotypically conventional family in Watford, Hertfordshire, and like a great many people I was eventually sent to school. However, my first coherent memory is of the day nursery I was placed in at the age of two. My mother, Pat, was in hospital having problems with her second pregnancy; my brother, Steve. My father, Reg, being at work all day in a local factory I had my first experience of a state institution and of rebelling against it.

I hated the fucking place. As soon as I got there at nine o'clock every morning, the jailers would sit me behind a table with the other kids and give me a small plastic car or other toy to play with for the next hour. I was bored senseless and I couldn't sit still obediently, which led to chastisement. Later, at eleven in the morning, the staff would put us all to bed for an hour and expect us to pretend to sleep on canvas sheets stretched between metal poles. I'd only been awake a few hours and felt restless. Any signs of movement were met with a telling off, or occasionally a smack from one of the prison officers. Fortunately, I can't remember what the rest of the day was like.

There were tender moments during this period as well. I probably gave my father hell by complaining about his cooking skills, which were inferior to those of my mother. He compensated for this by buying me a small toy each day, usually a matchbox car that he could ill afford. Also, an owl was living in the tree at the end of the back garden at the time, and it hooted a lot.

A previous, less coherent memory is of watching something like *Top of the Pops* with Mabel, my paternal grandmother, in 1965. I loved the vocal harmonies featured in at least one of the songs, but can't remember which song it was.

Compared to many, if not most of my friends now, my childhood was a bed of roses. Relatively speaking, I wasn't badly abused, though it didn't always feel like that at the time. I was no angel when I was a kid, but I never did anything unspeakably bad either. I was continually in trouble at school for minor misdemeanours – speaking out of turn, boisterousness, a short attention span, attention-seeking, hyperactivity – and the teachers encouraged my parents to mimic their own punitive actions, making family life difficult. I felt for many years that there was nowhere to turn without adults telling me off. On top of that I was a target for bullies in my age group. In particular the school bully, Tim Reynolds, was jealous of my perceived academic abilities, and he was encouraged by his vicariously competitive mother to compete with and undermine me. I felt socially awkward and felt that the other kids thought I was plain weird.

Aged eleven, I ended up at Watford Boys' Grammar School. Most people there came from the posh parts of town like the Cassiobury Estate and Bushey. Myself and Reynolds, the bully, were unusual there in terms of being residents of Garston, a relatively poor part of Watford. I wasn't as articulate as my peers, my home life featuring at times dysfunctional communication, and I had trouble being accepted by the other children. However, I developed a skill which is a tried and tested method of helping to deflect bullying: humour. I felt alienated, and after four years of it I began playing truant regularly. This would involve putting on my uniform to make my parents think I was going to school, then I'd go somewhere else. Often this was to avoid being bullied. More importantly it was a way simply to avoid the whole drag of being at school. Sometimes I would visit the local library where I could sit and read course material, as I wanted to pass the exams without the undue hassle of lessons. More often, I was drinking, taking drugs and getting tied up with the local and wider music scenes, within which I began to realise that there were many people out there who shared my sense of alienation. I also became attracted to the glamour and squalor of political radicalism, hanging out once a week at the Autonomy Centre set up in Wapping by anarchist punk band Crass and, when that closed down, at its successor, the Centro Iberico, a disused school in Westbourne Park squatted by Spanish syndicalist civil war veterans, which has since been demolished to make way for luxury flats. As was the case with many of my generation, politics and the immediate aftermath of punk somehow both vindicated and gave expression to the outsidership I was feeling.

My brother Steve was a source of support during this time. Watford Boys' Grammar School sent letters to my parents asking where I was; he helped intercept them so that I could forge letters back saying that I was ill. I didn't want to upset my parents, and in truth I was scared of my mother, whose frequent bad moods I had learned to absorb.

This was from 1980 to 1983, a great time to rebel and create because a youth culture then existed which lent itself to these impulses. With friends I put out around fifty punk fanzines during this period, and set up the avant-garde punk band the Godless Pinkoes – who were rubbish – with Ian Butler and Adam Penwarden from my school. Duncan Brown, later in Milk and Stereolab, also helped. Our first gig, in 1981, saw us opening the show at a community centre headlined by the Door and the Window, with Mark Perry on drums. This was the first time I ever met him. The show also featured the first ever post-Swell Maps performance by the great Nikki Sudden, whose lead guitarist on the night, Alan Tyler, badly burnt his hand whilst trying to imitate Nikki's useful trick of being able to sing, play guitar and smoke a fag all at the same time.

A Watford-based reactionary, Ian 'Sparky' Harrison, not only ran a local music equipment shop, Voxtrot: he also ran the Hertfordshire and Bedfordshire branch of the Musicians' Union, which insisted that musicians shouldn't perform unless each band member was paid the mandatory minimum rate of £40 per time. This was unrealistic for the Godless Pinkoes and all of the other decent Watford punk bands, the best of which were the Soft Drinks, the S-Haters and Rudimentary Peni. In any case, we believed that the best rock'n'roll has never been created by pro-

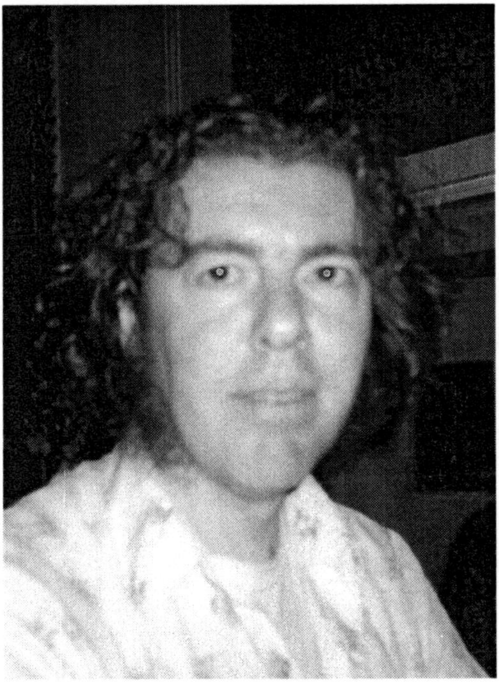

Alan Tyler

fessional jobsworths, but by kids primarily intent on amusing themselves.

'Sparky' organised a series of events which comprised the Herts and Beds rock competition. It had heats, semi-finals and then a final, the winning band ending up with the prize of a single out on EMI and some amplifiers. The Godless Pinkoes entered this for a laugh and performed a very well-received set at the Verulam Arms in St. Albans Road in one of the early heats, in front of our fans, who far outnumbered the sad old hairy heavy metal blokes there to see the other fuckers competing with us on the same bill. In spite of going down much better than the headbanging 'proper musicians', who were all about fifteen years older than us, the judges made us fourth out of five. The only reason we didn't come last was that Dave Greenfield, keyboard player with the Stranglers, was one of the judges and miraculously he was impressed by us. However, we were banned from ever playing at the venue again because our smoke effects had caused a fire and because apparently I'd provoked a fight with my allegedly inflammatory on-stage comments, setting headbangers and punk fans against each other. At the time I was sixteen years old and only five feet tall.

In order to wind up the local Musicians' Union further, I re-entered our band into the competition using a *nom de guerre*: the Acid Drops, named after the sweets I'd been throwing at the audience at the previous show to ham up the youth angle. Harrison fell for it and we turned up and performed. However, most

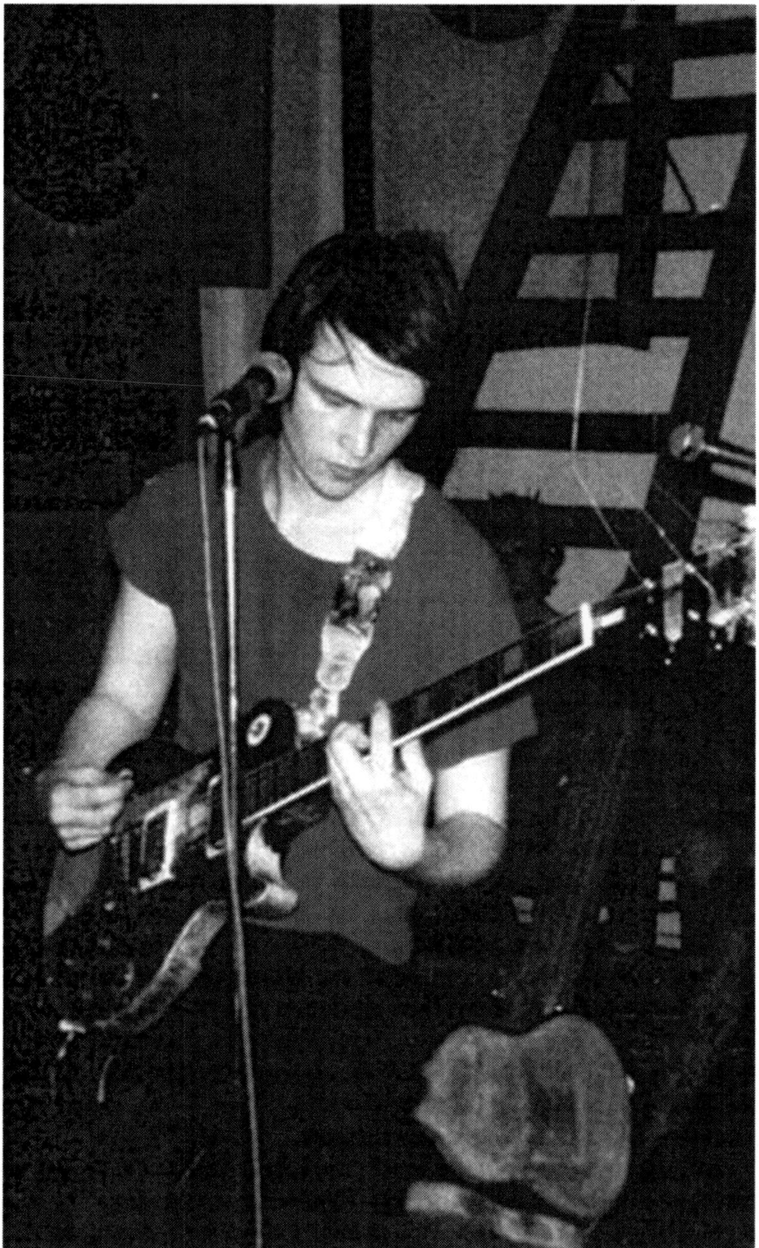

Nick Blinko, Rudimentary Peni, Wapping Autonomy Centre, 1982

of our fans, not realising we were playing, didn't show up, leaving us to play to a handful of headbangers. Harrison arranged for some of them to attack us after the show and we duly received a good kicking.

The following night, Harrison's shop, Voxtrot, was mysteriously fire-bombed, destroying most of the musical equipment inside and threatening the life of Harrison's dad, who lay asleep in the flat upstairs plugged into his dialysis machine. The next morning, two policemen came to my house to question me, alarming my parents. Under interrogation I was threatened with the twin charges of arson and attempted murder. Fortunately for me, they couldn't produce any evidence connecting me directly to the bombing. In fact, I'd had nothing to do with it. It was my mate Simon. Nobody was prosecuted.

During this time I wrote for various music magazines in addition to my own fanzines. I met some of my favourite musicians – including Jackie Leven, Mark Perry, Nikki Sudden and Robert Wyatt – and began hanging around and sometimes collaborating with those who I got on with. These also included talented musicians and songwriters who lived in or near to Watford, like Kieron O'Neill from the S-Haters, Nick Blinko from Rudimentary Peni, Tristan Garel-Funk from Sad Lovers and Giants, and Martin 'Drooper' Cooper from the Soft Drinks. Some of these characters, together with the company I kept at the anarchy centres, helped form my initiation into the murky world of 'mental illness'.

But in fact this initiation had begun earlier, courtesy of my grandfather, who had senile dementia. He had this routine of getting up early every Saturday morning, sharpening the pointed end of his umbrella, and performing sentry duty outside the local branch of Woolworths. He thought he was still in the Second World War, when the chip shop he ran had been bombed during the blitz. When the staff arrived for work, he'd threaten them with his lethal brolly and the old bill would be called; my dad had to collect his father from the police station on a weekly basis until finally the old geezer was carted off to the bin.

Alf Dellar, whose wife had predeceased him, also had a pile of sandbags outside his flat to protect him from attacks by the Germans. He'd often threaten my dad and other family members with knives, not recognising them. I was very fond of the bloke.

After he was sectioned into the psychogeriatric unit, he kept escaping and then being caught and brought back. Remarkably athletic for a man in his eighties, he was frequently able to outrun the young nurses chasing after him. Once, he tried to evade them by running up an alleyway which sadly led to a dead end, but luckily there was a pile of bricks at the end of the alleyway, allowing him to keep the nurses at bay for a while by lobbing them at them.

During the summer of 1983 I relocated with a few friends to Eastbourne, where we lived in a dole hostel and smoked huge quantities of cannabis. At the time 'Junior Wimbledon' was on in town, and my mate Dave Shann was considered the most talented young tennis player in Britain. He stayed with us for a time whilst attempting to win the tournament. Tennis is a posh sport, and middle and upper class players get corporate sponsorship, expensive rackets, and smart hotels to stay in. Dave, with his battered leather jacket with 'Danger Mouse' scrawled across the back, his pen and ink tattoos and his black and yellow cropped hair like a bumblebee, had none of these advantages: staying with us was a step up from the bushes and derelict barns to which he was accustomed.

A few hours after a serious drinking and smoking session lasting until five o'clock in the morning, it was the semi-final of Junior Wimbledon and Dave was pitched against a German whose racket, unlike Dave's, was unflawed: no strings missing, no holes, perfectly tuned, the lot. Dave was ahead on sets before eventually being disqualified for calling the umpire a cunt.

Angels With Dirty Faces

My bedroom had been seriously trashed. The posters had all been ripped from the walls, torn, screwed up and thrown haphazardly across the carpet. The drawers had all been pulled from the furniture and left upended, their contents scattered, some shredded into halves or quarters, the rest simply a disordered mess. Record sleeves had been ripped in two, especially those by bands like the Pop Group and Rudimentary Peni whose chosen images may have been perceived by normal people to be a bit controversial. Magazines had been rendered unreadable; books had been destroyed, crumpled pages of them littered all around. Clothes languished in awkward, random piles, pockets pulled out of trousers, interiors exposed like they'd been searched – which indeed they had. The bed was a foot from the wall, its mattress askew. A forensic expert looking at the scene would have concluded that either I'd lost the plot badly, or else there had been a major burglary.

In fact, the room had been trashed by my parents.

I was sixteen and it was 1981. I'd arrived home late in the afternoon from school, or from pretending to be at school, to find that my mum had searched my chest of drawers and came across two recent articles I'd written which she disliked. The shouting and screaming from my mum, though routine, was horrific and left me trembling like a jelly. By now she'd forbidden me from writing anything that wasn't connected to whatever I was supposed to be studying at school. She'd hidden both of the typewriters in the house, which meant that I had to go to friends' houses and use theirs when I wanted to knock out an article. Independent creativity was not simply frowned upon: in a secular way, it was evil.

I'd arranged that night to see the Jelly Babies, fronted by my friend the nascent Alan Tyler, and my dad had already kindly agreed to drive me and a couple of other kids from school to the show and back. The driving gave him an excuse to get out of the house. The school bully Tim Reynolds had turned up at the concert, his competitive attitude towards me making him worry that he could be missing out on something if I was there and he wasn't. I couldn't do anything without him trying to copy me or muscle in onto scenes I got involved with. He even made inept attempts at music journalism and organising a band, even though he shortly afterwards embarked on a career as a bank clerk. At the show, he came out with the routine verbal taunts and physical intimidation, and I have photographs to prove it; he was then at least twice my size. The drive back home to Garston was quiet and nervous, my father clearly as fearful of what would happen at the other end as I was.

The material devastation was there and no one spoke to each other, which in some ways was a relief. This bad atmosphere persisted through the next year and a half, as did my obsessive attempts to be creative. My identity burgeoned, but only under intense domestic pressure and hostility, and I was increasingly pathologised by those with greater power at the time. A nervous wreck, I stubbornly began to live my own life regardless, having to tell more and more lies to create the space for myself to do so.

"*I'm glad you're going*", my dad told me immediately before I left home for good and moved to Sussex University in 1983. He deserved a bit of peace and quiet for a change. Earlier he'd said: "*As soon as you get behind a typewriter, you turn into a nightmare.*" My mum had added: "*Things you write and make public when you're young, you don't realise, but it could be twenty or thirty years later and people can use it against you.*"

Actually, I've always found it to be the other way round. If you're a writer, even a bad one, and somebody treats you badly or behaves like a wanker in front of you, they may find decades later that something is written about them that leaves them trashed; it all comes back to haunt them. Writers tend to have long memories and the cunning to apply them, never letting things go. Anyway, it was time for me to move to Brighton.

My induction into the wacky world of 'mental illness' accelerated when I went to the University of Sussex, ostensibly to study. As a musician – albeit a poor one – and passable rock writer at the age of eighteen, I might have been expected to hang around with the trendiest kids in the hippest local scenes, with people who had hopes, dreams and ambitions. There were plenty of such characters around at Sussex University, and though it was clear that most of them would end up conventional, opportunities abounded for me to carry on where I'd left off culturally. Instead, I fell in with the likes of Adrian Chapman, Guy Delmistro, Pete Fleischmann, Hardman Hughes and Phil Murphy, all decent people whose lives were, or would soon become severely blighted by mental health problems, and the rock'n'roll took a back seat.

Three years of college flashed past in a blur of drink and drugs. Somehow I came out of it with a degree. In the process I helped run a project called Niteline, a nocturnal drop-in for depressed people and insomniacs which stayed open until six o'clock in the morning. I often organised the rota, sometimes staffing the place myself; essentially it was a place for people on the edge to hang about with and amuse each other, without normal people interfering. Most of the punters were mates of mine anyway, and it felt like a safe place.

A drug of choice for some time had been LSD, which led me to hang around with other people who also took too much of it: a bad move. In particular Charles Ross, the inspiration behind the character Trevor in my short story 'Homicide'[1], began to behave despicably as the hallucinogenics wore away at his ability to distinguish fantasy from reality. In his confusion, he became a serial stalker of women, all of whom were going out with blokes he'd befriended. Unsurprisingly this damaged his friendships. In 1987, at a time when I had the misfortune of living in a shared house on top of a big hill with the loser, he began to hit on my then-girlfriend Mina Sassoon really badly: there was no let-up for the months of him continually phoning her, writing deluded letters to her, following her in the street and hanging around outside her flat for hours on end, ringing the doorbell every few

1. Robert Dellar, 'Homicide', from *Suspect Device: A Reader in Hard Edged Fiction* ed. Stewart Home, Serpents Tail, 1998.

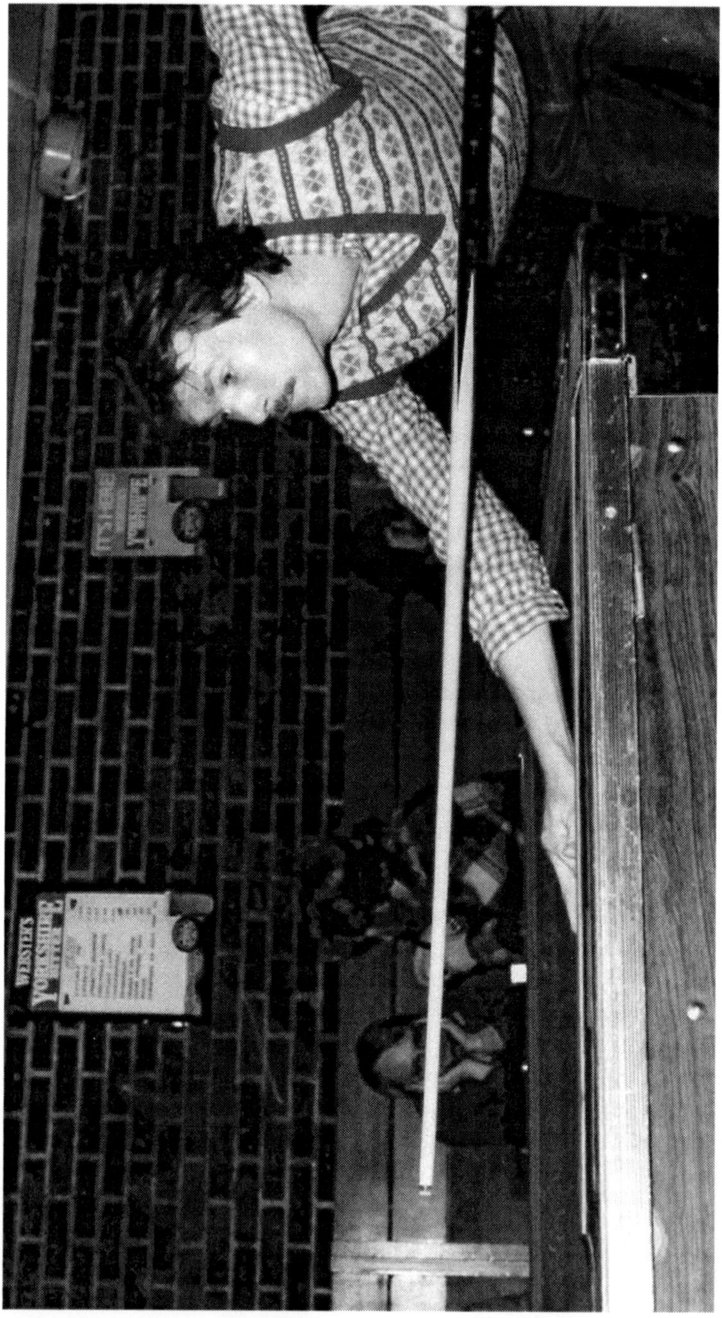

Hardman Hughes, Sussex University 1984

seconds. It was pretty scary, but what was equally scary was the blasé response of the people around me to Ross's behaviour. Nobody wanted to take it seriously until he did the same to them. Drugs and trendy half-baked anarchist ideas, I realised, had battered any sense of right or wrong out of many people around me, and not for the last time I felt the need to escape from the tired, low-life, sociopathic scene I'd become a part of.

We held a party one night at the shared house. Ross put thirty tabs of acid in the punch without telling anyone, mistakenly thinking that this would make it easier for him to pull, and leading to a few people becoming very distressed. This was the last straw, and very soon after I saw to it that we no longer shared a house. I derived a wicked pleasure from watching his posh parents collecting all of his belongings as he left under duress, humiliated. He moved around the corner into a squat with some of my other acquaintances. One of them, Steve Lockwood, had been threatening to torch a building for some months, figuring that society had it coming. Most of us thought he'd target a post office, as he held a particular grudge against the British postal system. However he decided instead to torch his own squat, destroying his and his friends' possessions in the process, leaving a large Victorian building completely gutted. Things like this seemed normal at the time. Steve's friends were initially a little annoyed with him, but they prided themselves in their broad-mindedness and soon forgave him. Steve was an interesting guy: his main interests involved drinking and gambling. Once, he'd married a woman in his native Bristol, and had convinced her that he was gainfully employed. He thought that he could pretend to go to work and spend office hours at the bookies, where he'd make enough money to generate a weekly wage packet. However, when the supposed payday arrived he was forced to come clean and his wife soon left him.

Some of my friends in Brighton were, in fact, engaged in more useful activities, even if none of these extended to day-jobs. In 1985, Phil Murphy formed the Regular Guys, one of the greatest rock bands to emerge from this country during that decade. Mingling slow, moody ballads and complex three-part harmonies with lewd, Stooges-style wild man rock'n'roll, they were head, shoulders and torso above every other band in town. Emerging as they did from a low-life scene helped them sabotage themselves, and they failed to achieve the success they deserved: their lyrics, which made Joy Division sound like pop funsters Madness, probably didn't help. Other bands I liked included power-pop trio Salad From Atlantis and avant-garde proto-grunge quintet the Unbelievables, but remarkably for a town containing so many musicians there was very little else, which in part explained my loss of interest in writing about music around that time. Brighton indie bands like Blow Up and 14 Iced Bears weren't bad and were doing well, but after the explosion of ideas, experimentation and intensity in the immediate wake of punk, formulaic guitar-pop, however well-intentioned, felt like something of a let-down.

In 1984, Phil Murphy, myself and one or two others had run a magazine at college called *Nice Try But it Won't Work*. This was in response to the middle-class, self-consciously intellectual and theatrically right-on people who got on our nerves when we lived on campus at Sussex University. *Nice Try*, which ran weekly without fail for nine issues, was a great opportunity to wind people up, and it ran articles on pool, football, snooker and telly programmes such as *Minder*. Our editorial policy excluded words with more than two syllables and sentences containing more than ten words as we deconstructed and copied the most basic tabloid journalism. The rag became an instant cult classic.

Much of our invective was aimed at Brighton Labour Briefing. Phil, myself and most of our friends had chosen Sussex as the university to attend mainly due to its radical, far-left reputation, looking for the spirit of rebellion. I'd seen *Daily Mail* headlines saying something like 'don't let your child go to Sussex!' after a visiting David Owen was pelted with eggs and rotten fruit by student radicals, and thought *"that sounds good, I'll go there"*, as did many others. However, the university Students Union seemed to be controlled by people who'd mastered politically sound language and reached earnest, sometimes gratuitously awkward positions on serious issues which were grasped only in abstraction. It seemed fake and we knew most of them would grow out of it. Further, the zealots at Briefing, in charge of the Union, seemed intensely motivated by personal power and used their enhanced political awareness as a tool to bully and control the less enlightened masses on campus. In a twisted way it was as if they were the ruling class and we were the proletariat. All dissent was disallowed. Ordinary students bowed to or avoided the likes of Janice Turner, Alick Bridger, Fiona Morton and Bryn Griffiths like school kids scared of their headmaster. You could spot these guardians of our conscience a mile off. The women wore burka-type clothes all day as a feminist statement, while the men minced along the high street in dungarees, waving carrier bags saying 'the Body Shop'. As well as continually putting the boot in on these hacks in the pages of *Nice Try*, alarming them to the extent that they tried to ban it, we used to regularly mess up their meetings. Bryn Griffiths, subsequently a low-ranking trade union official, once announced: *"If any of these* Nice Try *bastards try to disrupt our meeting, they'll be out – through the window if necessary!"* A hollow threat. Taken as a group, we were far harder and more streetwise than the young entryists.

These prefects were scared of people who were 'mentally ill', often dismissing disordered, psychotic behaviour as evidence of the inherent 'fascism' of those exhibiting it if their political positions differed. The issue of madness was inextricably linked to the bitter disputes which took place between Briefing and, over its short duration, *Nice Try*, the contents of which often reflected the fact that many of its contributors were seriously losing the plot. This episode permanently altered my priorities and was good experience for what lay ahead.

After university finished I spent a year in Brighton on the dole, putting out the fanzine *Straight Up* and doing a bit of voluntary advice work, but generally going nowhere. Unlike many of my associates then, I was dissatisfied with this. Mina got a job in Leytonstone as a nursing assistant and I followed her up to East London where we lived for a few weeks in a small room at the nurses' home. Some of the Brighton crew decided that they too wished to relocate themselves to London, and so it was that Pete Fleischmann and myself found ourselves wandering along Grove Green Road, pre-M11, one afternoon in broad daylight with a crowbar.

There were several empties along this stretch of the route of the planned motorway. The first few houses we broke into weren't right; they were burnt out, or else clearly earmarked for new tenants. Eventually we arrived at 113 Grove Green Road, E11. It looked all right. As we began trying to get the front door off with the crowbar, the next door neighbour came out and peered at us over the fence. *"What are you two doing?"* she enquired.

"We're homeless", we explained. *"We were looking along the street and this place looks empty, we want to see if it's worth squatting."*

"The place isn't in bad condition", she told us. *"The electricity's on and everything, but there's no need for you to break in. The back door's open, you can come through my house, hop over the garden fence and let yourselves in."*

It was great: a huge Victorian house in the middle of a long terrace, without mod cons and in disrepair, but for me at least, a happy home for nearly a year. Pete, Mina and myself were joined by Rachel Emmett, Tony Fisher and Matt Pratt from Brighton and, as has not often been the case in homes I've shared, the dynamics between us worked and things were fun: lots of gigs, drink, drugs and partying. One of the first things that happened was that a hook appeared sinisterly on the wall a foot above the pillow on Matt's bed. Matt claimed it had been there already, but he said that every time he moved into a new room; the truth was revealed when one of his girlfriends spilled the beans when she was drunk. Our time here was brought to an end in August 1988, inevitably by eviction. The night prior to this, we held a party and pop concert in the back garden, starring the Fish Brothers and the Astronauts. The former were at the time a sideline of Salad From Atlantis frontman Martin Cooper, a namesake of the erstwhile Soft Drinks singer, and they were a duo playing Victorian music hall and comedy punk. The Astronauts were a singularly intense, songwriterly folk-punk act from Welwyn Garden City: led by Mark Wilkins, by this time they'd already been in action for over a decade and released several fine albums. Earlier that day we'd forced open an electricity meter in the basement and it had been full of 50p coins from way back, which we used to pay the bands' expenses.

The Astronauts were on first, in front of a sizeable audience of Special Brew-swigging down-and-outs. Opening the set with 'Fatigue' from the band's album *All Done by Mirrors*, Mark appeared nervous as neighbours, some looking rather annoyed, peered from their windows as the sun went down. Then a few songs into the set, a pisshead from Welwyn decided to heckle the band incoherently. The guitarist, Tony, took exception and responded by laying into the heckler and kicking fuck out of the bastard. Myself and others dived in and broke it up before anyone was badly hurt; however, Tony had forgotten to remove his guitar before this altercation, and the instrument was battered to pieces. Both the guitar and its player were too shaken by the incident to continue. Fortunately, the Astronauts were experienced profes-

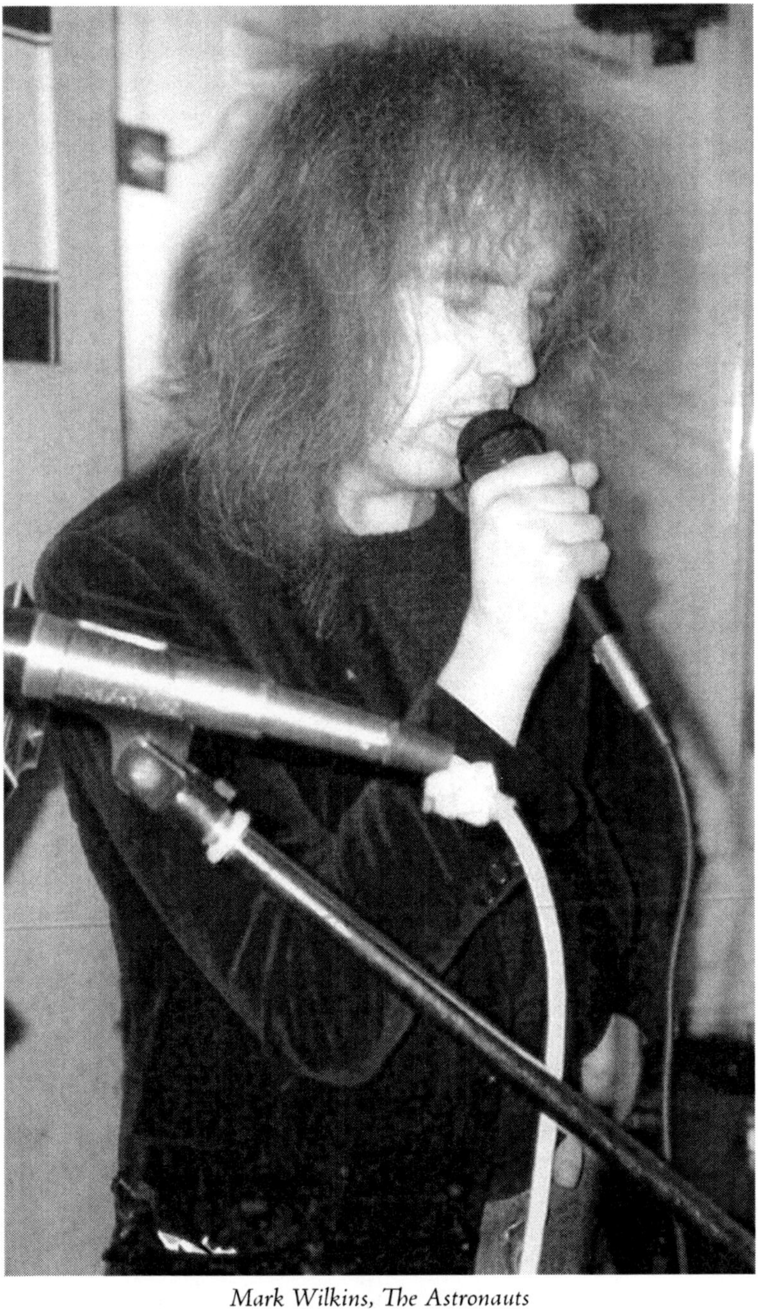

Mark Wilkins, The Astronauts

sionals and had a reserve guitarist standing in the wings in case something like this happened. The bloke pulled on the number twelve shirt and the show resumed. Due to neighbours complaining about the noise and the big bonfire at the end of the garden, the night was frequently interrupted by visits from the police and fire brigade, but somehow we repeatedly managed to get rid of them. It wasn't until eleven the following morning, when the bailiffs arrived, that the party finished. Fortuitously, this was when the pubs opened. Twenty of us trotted off to the Northcote, a stereotypical East London geezers' boozer. This being prior to licensing law reforms, we drank there until 2.30 in the afternoon: chucking out time.

The landlord intercepted me as we left, apparently identifying me as a ringleader. We'd had problems at this pub before because many of the locals were prejudiced against squatters, and we'd been kicked out a few times for minor indiscretions such as sitting on the floor, and asking to be served snakebite. It would be a year or two before the whole street became full of squatters as rent-payers were moved out in preparation for the M11. The landlord was agitated. *"I don't want to see you, or your mates, in here ever again! Right?"* he hollered.

"What, have we done something to upset you?" I asked. I thought we'd been on our best behaviour.

"Well, look at the fucking state of the lot of you!" he blasted.

After we moved out, other people we knew squatted the house briefly and they too were evicted. The council then sent along a crew to trash the place: they literally sawed all of the stairs and floorboards out, so that if you looked through the front door, which had in fact been replaced by a thick concrete wall, you'd have seen a sheer drop to the cellar deep below. And a perfectly good house was left gutted and uninhabited for a number of years before finally it was demolished to make way for the motorway. When road protesters subsequently took over the street, a plaque appeared outside reading *"This House Was Once Somebody's Home"*.

It was mine when in December 1987 I began working for mental health charity Mind in Hammersmith as an outreach worker on the Community Programme, a Thatcherite initiative to help the long-term unemployed back to work and bring down the dole figures, in those days officially around three million. Community Programme jobs were usually for sixteen hours a week, ostensibly had a training element, and paid fifteen quid more than the dole.

The training accompanying this job involved induction into psychodynamic theory, mainly Freud, Winnicott and Klein, and I read what I was told to conscientiously. I've no objection to these theories as models, and at times they can be useful and hold true, but I dispute the notion that these teachings describe universal truth. As far as philosophy and psychology are concerned, I've always held that it's best to take a bit here, a bit there, as and when it's useful, without regarding any particular model as biblical. For example, Freud's 'Oedipus complex' may have been a way of understanding elements of Charles Ross's stalking, but for most of us it would have at most marginal significance. However, it would have been heretical to say that to my bosses at Mind in Hammersmith, well-intentioned folk though they were.

For the productive part of my job I had three 'clients' who I visited weekly in their homes, 'befriending' them within strict guidelines and being encouraged to use psychodynamic techniques on them – a potentially dangerous activity when the practitioner's psychoanalytic skills are only very basic. I was aware of my limitations and didn't go over the top with the mind games; I knew that I was almost the only person that these three clients would speak with each week and didn't wish to make them more confused than they already were. It was debatable whether any of these three really had 'mental health problems' in any conventional sense. One was an elderly, anxious woman whose main problem seemed to be loneliness, and she appreciated my company once a week as somebody she could talk to without being patronised. Another was an elderly man who simply wasn't coping due to extremely low intelligence. Shunned by the public, he too appreciated my company. He spent most of his meagre welfare benefits at the bookies and tried to disguise this by claiming he'd been mugged all the time. In a sense I felt privileged to spend time with these marginalised people, and I hope they saw it the same way too, but if I'd tried 'analysing' them it would only have wound them up.

The third client was an Irishman in Fulham with no memory, and what I would now call chronic agoraphobia. What would be the point of practicing psychoanalytic techniques on someone who can't even remember their own name from one day to the next, let alone mine? Mind in Hammersmith encouraged me to do precisely that. The bloke accepted my company as a positive thing and had a vague visual recognition of me over consecutive visits, but couldn't recall threads of conversation. I never worked out what the amnesia was all about, but in retrospect it would have been more useful if I'd employed the traditional, pragmatic psychiatric-model techniques of combating agoraphobia: encouraging him to push the boundaries, get out of bed and go a few feet further each time, calming and reassuring him as he took these steps. Having said this, he may well have got lost, and in any case this wasn't what I was advised to do.

"You'll never go far in the helping profession" predicted my external supervisor, a psychoanalyst who thought I had an attitude problem. I'd missed or been late for a few appointments with him, basically because I thought he was full of shit and had nothing useful to say, and he pathologised this: *"You seriously need to work on yourself if you're not to be a failure all your life."* I daresay that my attitude problem has had a greater impact on the helping profession than anything done by this twerp before or since.

There was also a celebrity group supervisor, lording it up in front of the whole gang of Community Programme outreach workers. His name, not inappropriately: Jo Berke, the famous associate of R.D. Laing from the 1960s. If he hadn't been a mate of Laing's nobody would ever have heard of him, but in the event he became renowned for his work with his 'client' Mary Barnes at Kingsley Hall, Laing's infamous East End therapeutic community where people were allowed and even encouraged to 'go mad', live and work through their madness and come out the other side, sadder but wiser. In the late sixties, Barnes used to cover herself from head to toe in her own excrement all day, howl a lot and generally make herself a nuisance to the other community residents. Berke was her therapist, and although he became exasperated and assaulted her a few times, she became a little better after a few years, did some painting and wrote a few poems. In fact the two of them wrote a book together about their interaction, and it became a best-seller in Laing's slipstream.

I wasn't impressed with Jo Berke. During the group supervision sessions in his posh flat in Primrose Hill, in the course of which his pet rabbit would hop around the living room, he'd offer very few constructive observations or pieces of advice, choosing instead to revel in his imaginary star trip. He nearly lost the gig by hitting on Karen, the best looking female out of the crew of long-term unemployed being helped back to work. He made sick jokes about incest, *"keeping it all in the family"* and other such side-splitters, completely unmindful of how the workers' lives may have been affected and blighted by this issue. Mostly he just spent the sessions talking about himself.

We were paid very little, but a perk of the job was a London-wide travelcard which, given my poverty at the time, would have been useful. Using the cheque Mind in Hammersmith had given me, I bought mine at Leyton tube ticket office: it was meant to last for a year. But when I used this card on the East London Docklands railway line, it transpired that the card had been filled in incorrectly by the ticket office staff, leading London Transport to confiscate it and suggest, wrongly, that I'd forged it, an impression abetted by the staff's apparent denial that they'd sold me the ticket, which suggested to me that they may have been onto some kind of scam themselves.

A London Transport investigator, 'Bob' Rumfitt, knocked at my squat at seven in the morning and I answered. I led him to the kitchen, people being asleep in all of the other rooms. We had an interesting kitchen. It was filthy. There was a hole in the ceiling through which the bathroom upstairs was visible, allowing the leak from the cistern, as well as piss if anyone missed the bowl, to drip through onto the sink and the abundant unwashed dishes. There was also a problem with mice, and every morning there'd be a hollowed-out loaf of bread into which the small furry creatures, which had cute little round ears and noses that twitched, had nocturnally burrowed, leaving only the crust and a pile of droppings inside. It must have been quite unlike any other kitchen 'Bob' had ever seen and he took a dislike to me immediately. The upshot of our crack-of-dawn meeting was that I was threatened with prosecution for fraud.

Two weeks later, 'Bob' and a colleague came to Mind in Hammersmith, the location being at my insistence, to threaten me further. As back-up, I made sure that my bosses were there, though I suspect that they too may have thought I'd been up to something. Initially, the London Transport scum promised court action and the likelihood of a £2,000 fine, a fortune for me at the time. After some gentle-voiced negotiation from the bosses and sarcasm from me, a compromise was reached whereby my card was confiscated and I had to pay a small on-the-spot fine, with the promise that if I was ever in trouble with London Transport again they'd throw the book at me. Mind never replaced the travelcard.

Karen, who Jo Berke had failed to pull, was an interesting woman. Heavily into Wilhelm Reich, she believed his theories about 'orgone', a life force which infuses all living organic matter and which is light blue in colour if seen through a certain lens that Reich had invented. The theory went that, if you sat inside an orgone accumulator on top of a range of mountains, it would cure cancer and generally give you a sense of well-being. This machine was a box made out of lead, lined on the inside and outside with rotting vegetables or other organic matter. If, however, you sat inside such a box in the city, for example on a crowded tube platform, it would have the reverse effect and unleash Deadly Orgone Radiation. Reich also thought he could make it rain with his cloud-busting machine, and Karen believed this too. She said she could literally see the Deadly Orgone Radiation at London Bridge tube each day on the way to work. Other Mind in Hammersmith workers also held strange beliefs, often due to swallowing Freudian concepts too uncritically. When I said I had two cats, one woman remarked: *"of course, the reason people like cats is because they unconsciously remind them of pubic hair, especially from the birth experience"*.

The outreach project was cut short in August 1988 when it lost its funding at very short notice, giving us inadequate time to prepare our clients for the withdrawal of the service, Thatcher having decided to pull the Community Programme. After nine months of sometimes fascinating but conceptually flawed work, I was briefly back on the dole and homeless, the eviction having occurred around the same time. I skippered for a few weeks, then got a job with Mind in Croydon.

Mind in Croydon was a nice middle-class outfit befitting the area. It had been set up by the elderly philanthropist Nora Croft, who'd installed her daughter-in-law Margot as director. Well-meaning blue-rinsers ran the show from top to bottom. At the time the Club, a detached house located in Altyre Road which ran between East Croydon train station and the Fairfield Halls venue, was financed by profits from Mind in Croydon's shop in affluent Purley, although the club has since attracted statutory funding. You could get kitted out cheaply and smartly at the Mind charity shop: honestly, you'd be amazed by some of the stuff that rich people chuck out. The club ran according to a paternalistic, pitying model of mental health care which even in 1988 was becoming anachronistic. Established in 1971, the club had institutionalised dozens of local fruits within its walls.

The idea was that the club was a family. The fruits were children, the staff were parent figures. To this end, the day-to-day management of the place required a couple, who would get five grand a year each and a rent-free flat in the attic at the top of the house. Seeing the job up for grabs in a *Guardian* advertisement and at a loss for where to go after the eviction, Mina and myself jointly applied. It was irresponsible of Mind in Croydon's management to employ us, given that we were both only 23 and lacked experience relevant to a task of the magnitude of running a large, busy day centre accommodating up to a hundred fruits a day. But because of the low remuneration, they weren't spoilt for choice. A lesbian couple had applied who for all I know may have had the skills required, but somehow I think a same-sex couple would have threatened the assumptions implicit in Mind in Croydon's vision of social care. Our paperwork and interview were OK. We were in.

Many of the more charismatic fruits attending the club were, ironically, lesbians, who turned up in spite of the homophobia rampant amongst the other fruits, who were mostly fallen from middle-class backgrounds and to a large extent Christians, who held the belief that homosexuality was an airborne transmitted disease like influenza. I have fond memories of drunken nights out with Brenda Carter and her mates, who wound up the straights by shouting *"look at the arse on that chick!"* and suchlike at women standing at the bar, to widespread confusion and disapproval. They were worse than blokes working on building sites. A fair few chicks at the club came out during our two years in Croydon, encouraging the contagion theory. Mina and myself stuck up for the lesbians making, I thought, the management feel very awkward.

Among many other fruits I liked were David Hardcastle, who during his mad phases would inform me and Mina that we were destined to go to hell for not being married, and Peter Barker, an elderly alcoholic who we unbarred from the place when we started working there. Peter was judged and looked down upon by other fruits, who couldn't understand how someone of his clear intelligence would 'choose' to spend his life drunk. He often forgot that he'd moved flat, and wondered why the keys didn't work

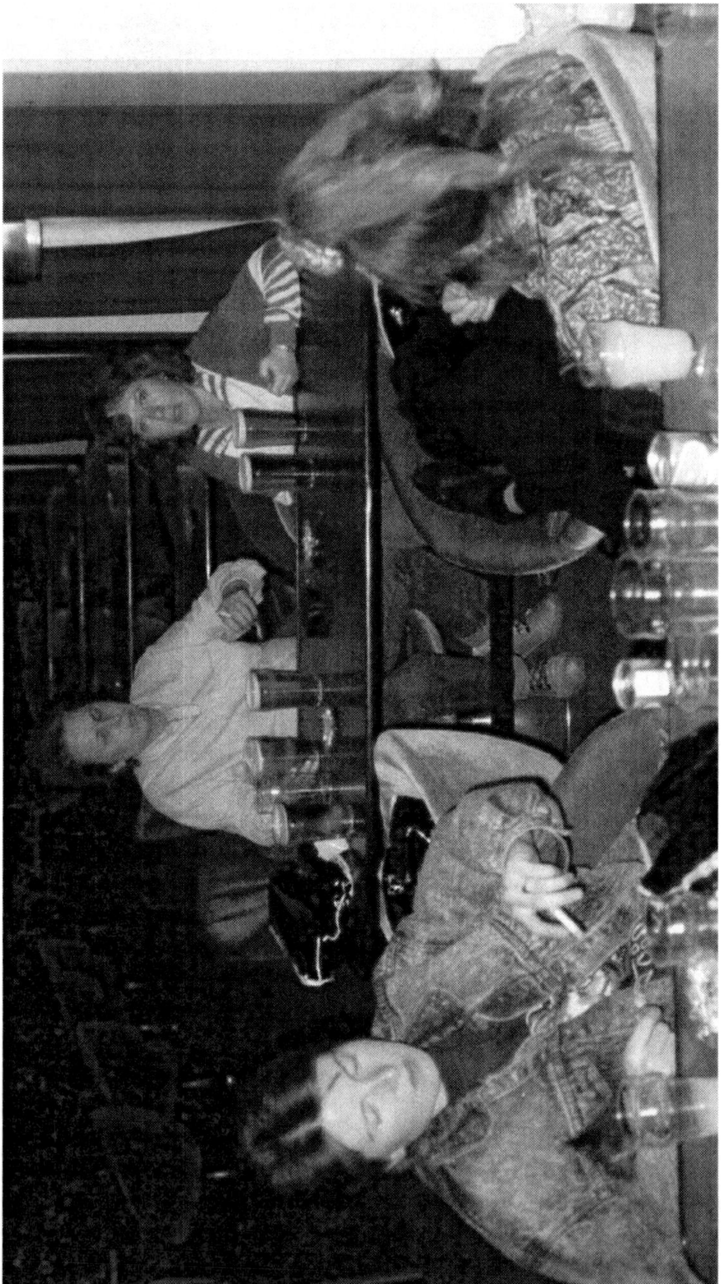

Fairfield Club regulars

when he tried to let himself into one of his old places after a session. He'd been traumatised by his experiences as an adolescent soldier in Africa in the Second World War. On the one occasion in his life when he'd declined to take a drink when offered, it turned out that the bottles had been sabotaged by the enemy, contaminated with minute fragments of glass, and his mates died; Peter felt somehow responsible. I've come to know dozens of ex-squaddies since, and almost without exception they've emerged from the army emotionally damaged. Peter lived on cider and his considerable wits before dying during the 1990s.

The fruits were mostly decent, but on the whole the spirit at the club was one of resigned, abject despair. Many had been attending since its inception and were part of the furniture on which they sat all day, quiet, subjugated and still. It was like a hospital-from-home. The slightest change in routine was seen as catastrophic. At the beginning of our stewardship of this dump, two speakers from Alcoholics Anonymous had been scheduled to visit and give an evening talk. When this overran by five minutes, fruits flocked to the canteen counter extremely agitated, complaining that their night-time hot chocolate was late. Meanwhile, the UK mental health survivors' movement was starting to take off.

Strands of radicalism around the mental health scene have threaded through centuries, but in modern form became notable only during the 1960s in the work of 'anti-psychiatrists' encompassing too vast a political spectrum to truly cohere as a movement; and none of it was fruitcake-led. Most of the movers and shakers had in fact trained, and continued to practice as doctors. Writers and activists such as R.D. Laing and David Cooper approached the subject from the left, whereas others, notably Thomas Szasz, opposed psychiatric orthodoxy from a far-right, 'stand on your own two feet' perspective. This came at a time when psychiatry had been granted new status and a raft of new powers, enshrined in the 1958 Mental Health Act, following the introduction of a range of psychiatric pharmaceuticals from the mid-1950s: drugs which suppressed symptoms associated with psychosis at the expense of making the fruits taking them physically ill. The link between the pharmaceutical industry and psychiatric practice, thus established, would persist and indeed intensify over the years as capitalism developed new and more advanced techniques to consolidate itself. The 'medical model' prevailed, treating mental distress as an 'illness' with unproven yet taken-as-fact genetic and biochemical causes, and generally overlooking the demonstrable social determinants of experiences and behaviours labelled as madness. Psychiatry increasingly became a method of social control. From 1970 and heavily influenced by Laing and his contemporaries, self-help and campaigning groups like the Mental Patients Union and CAPO (Campaign Against Psychiatric Oppression) were set up to challenge this, taking explicit anti-psychiatry stances, with fruits like Eric Irwin, Frank Bangay and Julian Barnett issuing manifestos, performing their poetry, wearing sandwich-boards in the street and laying the foundations of what would mutate into the 'user movement'.

Building on this grass-roots agitation, during the 1980s mental health activists like Peter Campbell, Alan Leader, Kathy Pelikan and Louise Pembroke organised themselves in various permutations using different group names: most significantly Survivors Speak Out, who used the media and negotiation with professionals as well as much behind-the-scenes debate to bring mental health rights issues to a public previously unaware that such issues existed. They largely dispensed with the crude and reductive notion that doctors deliberately set out to worsen their patients' lives, instead appealing to people's compassionate and humanitarian instincts, and it was a huge step forward paving the way for the later explosion of user-led activity into the mainstream. It wasn't perfect: too much time was wasted arguing about terminology and engaging in personal power struggles. But ground-breaking movements are never perfect, there being no template to measure performance against, making trial and error often unavoidable. What is certain is that later groups like Mad Pride and Survivors Poetry, as well as developments such as mental health advocacy services and the statutory duty of service providers to consult with and involve service users in the planning, delivery and evaluation of services, would not have arisen as strongly as they did without the brave work of these committed and articulate pioneers.

None of which cut much ice with members of the Fairfield Club. At the time Mind in Camden was ran by a guy named David Hill, a clinical psychologist going through a radical phase. We invited a speaker from their user group to explain to Croydon users how they could organise and stick up for themselves, and

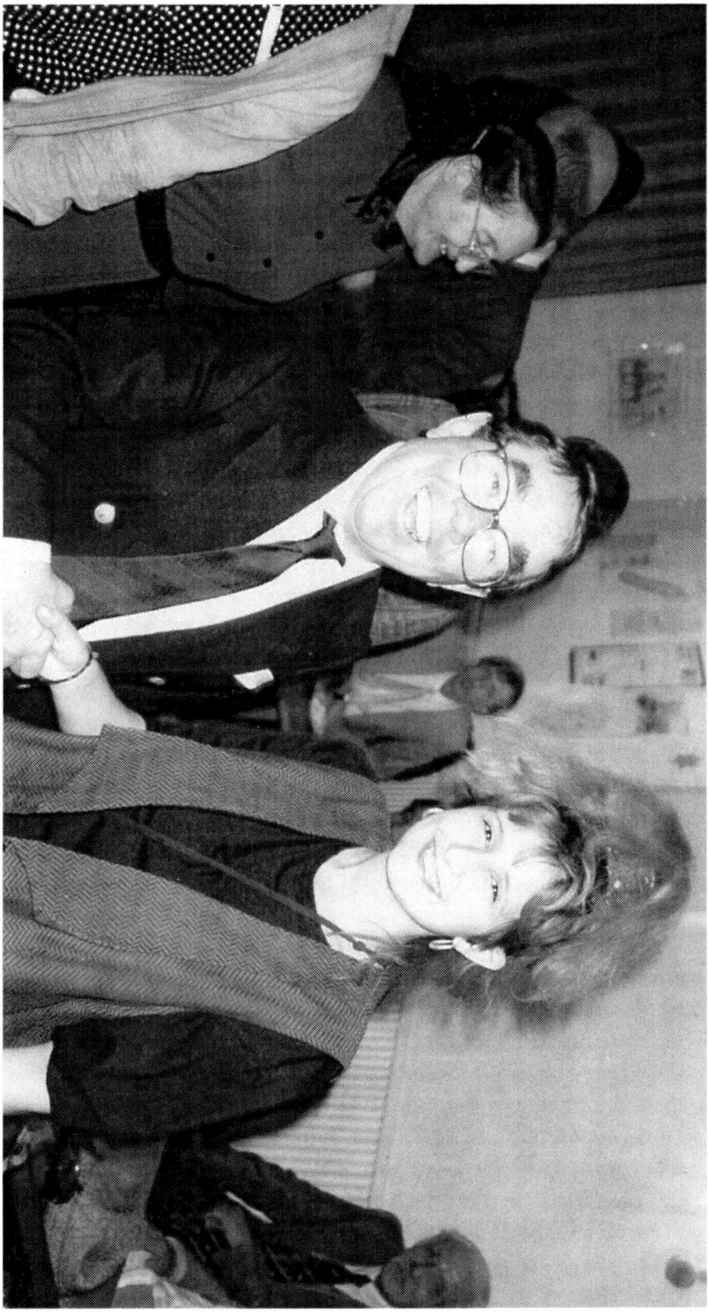

Ronnie Corbett and Mina Sassoon, The Fairfield Club, Croydon, 1990

maybe help make the world a better place for themselves and others like them. But basically the Fairfield Club folk's attitude was: *"Fuck off! We want our hot chocolate!"* Even the idea that mental health users could have meetings without paid professionals in attendance frightened them: they thought it would inevitably lead to a ruck. They were victims of taught dependency.

None of this was Ronnie Corbett's fault. It had been a tradition of the club to invite the local mayor to its anniversary celebration, and Mina and I oversaw its seventeenth. The mayor turned up with all his medallions and his Father Christmas outfit, stepped out of his Rolls Royce and swanned about regally. He ordered David Hardcastle to *"get out of that seat and find a job!"* He suggested to Mina that, instead of wasting her time helping psychiatric cases, she'd be better off getting a proper job in the tower block full of offices across the road. And then he was chauffeured back to the town hall after getting his butler to inspect his clothing for fleas. For the club's eighteenth birthday the following year, I insisted on getting a celebrity guest who lived locally, as opposed to the lord mayor. Patrick Moore being on tour in the then-apartheid South Africa, and various members of punk outfit the Damned being otherwise busy, Corbett had to do.

He was great. He spent all day wandering around the centre with his wife, who was twice his height, chatting to the characters, being in no way patronising, in what seemed a friendly and natural way with no obvious star-trip. OK, so he isn't funny on telly, but believe me, in real life the man is a star. He ended up donating thousands of pounds to the club to help keep it going. Respect to the bloke.

Out of boredom I reacquainted myself with musicians I'd known before moving to Brighton. Old friends like Alan Tyler and Duncan Brown were becoming successful, and they were chauffeured to their local pub in Camden every night in record-company sponsored limousines, with free cocaine, groupies and expensive designer clothes. The Camden scene back then centred around a pub called the Falcon, with nightly music concerts in its back room, and the best bands were playing there all the time: local new kids on the block like the Rockingbirds, Silverfish and th' Faith Healers, as well as established stars like Alex Chilton, Green On Red and Kevin Coyne, and it became something a regular haunt as I commuted from Croydon at every available

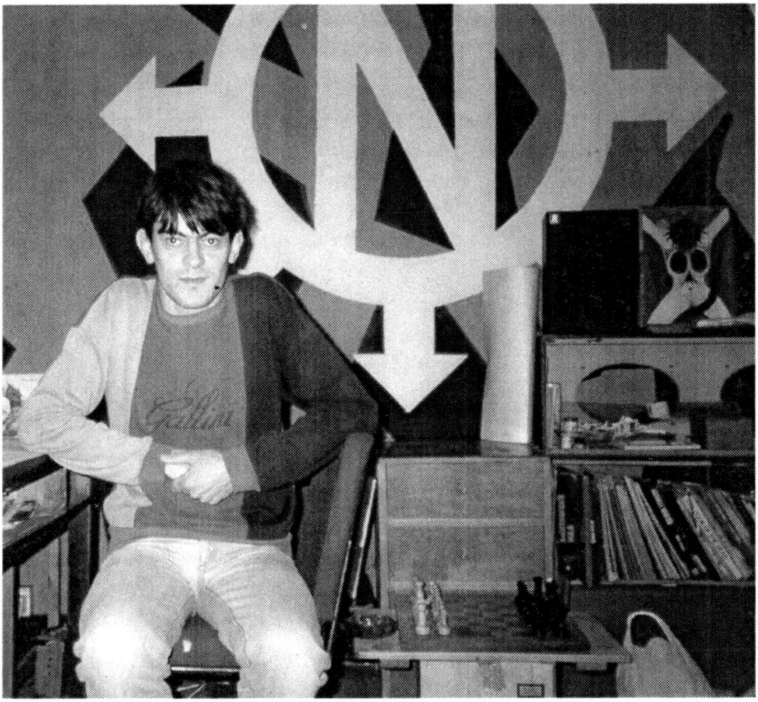

Andy Martin, The Apostles, Hackney, 1991

opportunity. Getting into the spirit, I booked the Fish Brothers from Brighton to play one evening at the Fairfield Club. Their singer Martin Cooper was mobbed by elderly women drunk on the punch we'd provided, and the band went down especially well with the alkies amongst the membership who enjoyed notable sing-alongs such as 'I'm A Drinker' and 'Down In One'. But outside the job there was nothing to do in Croydon and all real life was further north. I spent a lot of time in Hackney, hanging out a lot with Andy Martin and his sidekick Dave Fanning of anarcho-punk band the Apostles, and the evolving series of housemates they had in their dilapidated co-op place in Brougham Road, London Fields, a street full of psychedelic brightly-painted caravans, drug addicts, Autonomy Centre veterans and passing brew crew travellers. At first, the pair lived with a bunch of glue sniffers who once used a sledgehammer to demolish a supporting wall on the ground floor of the house while the musicians were out: consequently, when years later the co-op was requisitioned by the council and let out to more conventional tenants, Andy's place at the end of the terrace was the only one to be condemned and demolished.

I'd first met Andy at the Autonomy Centre in 1981, just after he'd formed his band. He seemed mad. I liked him. One evening, slogans like 'Andy Martin is a fucking queer' had been scrawled across the wall of the centre with a marker pen; Andy was almost in tears at the perceived affront, even though the graffiti was in what appeared to be his own handwriting. The Apostles went on to make around ten vinyl albums, thirty cassette releases and several singles including the indie hits 'Pigs For Slaughter' and 'Mob Violence', both of which promoted the joys of throwing bricks at the old bill, trashing posh cars, poisoning meat-eaters and mugging rich bastards. Poor musicianship and even worse studio productions rendered much of it unlistenable and the records fell short despite, I think, displaying the skills of a unique and talented songwriter. Andy could write prose too, and his special gift was for polemic. What the polemic was about didn't matter: he'd flit between anarchism, fascism, Leninism and respectable concerned citizenship but as a stylist he was always consistent. He was on fire all the time, so full of anger and bitterness, but always with residual optimism. The riffs and melodic hook-lines in his songs will always be etched into and resounding around my brain.

Meanwhile, Mina and myself left Mind in Croydon wishing neither ourselves nor the club to get stale. Beforehand we'd organised a few club holidays, most notably a fortnight in Klonakilty on the south coast of Ireland for twenty people. Glynn Davies drove us there in a bus all the way from Croydon, via Wales and a ferry. Years later he died by ploughing his car under a lorry on a motorway. Ireland went well, even when Glynn ran straight through a plate glass door in his chalet, having registered it only as a transparent space: the chalet owners were understanding, because, as it transpired, they too had 'long-term schizophrenia'. We couldn't get away from it.

Mina and I visited the club three times after we stopped working there. On the first occasion I watched the news on telly featuring Leonora, one of the holidaymakers we'd taken to Ireland, a lively, pretty young black woman who we got on with, being carted off, cuffed and chained by a dozen old bill. The next time,she was again on telly, being sentenced to life imprisonment, commuted to psychiatric hospital, for the murder of her six month old baby. I'm not making this up. The third and last time, the telly informed us that she'd escaped from hospital and thrown herself under a tube in Archway, a popular suicide location. It seemed like bad luck to go back again to the Fairfield Club, so we stopped. Leonora had stabbed her baby eighty times: there couldn't have been much left of the fucking thing.

Incidents like this, thankfully and contrary to common perception, are almost unheard of within the mental health community. I remember Leonora as a gentle, kind soul. She must have become very mad and been at her wits' end. I guess she couldn't live with it. It's bad when that happens.

Barbed Wire Halo

Our friend Tony Fisher helped us crack open the squat in Hackney, which was on the top floor of a four-storey block. Thick, strongly secured steel grilles covered the doors and windows to protect the place from people like us who may have wanted to live there, even though the flat had been empty for several years and was in severe disrepair, especially the roof. It took a lot of noise and brute force to get in, reattach the real front door which had been pulled off its hinges by the council and left lying in the living room, and change the locks. But this being the Pembury Estate, the neighbours, though curious, didn't seem to mind. One, an ex-squaddie, even came out of his flat and helped.

It was 1990. The roof had a very large hole in it, and whenever it rained, water came cascading through the ceiling. I installed a contraption in the attic consisting of ropes, buckets and bin liners to keep the flooding at bay. After a downpour I'd have to access the attic via a hatch in the ceiling of our next door neighbour Philippa Kerruish's flat and empty the buckets. The first time that I attempted this operation, I was freaked out by the hundreds of pigeons fluttering around my head in the dark. Not only had they made a home in the attic, they'd also commandeered a space in a boiler area up there as a cemetery, and piles of dead pigeons in various stages of decomposition lay on top of each other on and around the steel cylinder servicing part of the block. Soon, I realised that the pigeons were my friends, and they were more afraid of me than I was of them.

As well as Philippa – who we'd met in Croydon where she'd been working as a social worker and who had alerted us to the empty flat, aware that Mina and myself were homeless and skint – a few other interesting characters were scattered around the building. Andy Davey was one of the drug dealers on the block and I regularly scored from him. He was a disturbed but harmless loser who was later murdered by kids, who were never caught, on the forecourt outside the block – aged 35, according to the *Hackney Gazette*, on his way home from the Samuel Pepys after ten pints of lager.

Another Andy was Falklands Andy, so named because he'd served as a squaddie and weapons instructor in the South Atlantic. He'd squatted the flat next door to us on the opposite side to Philippa. He'd discharged himself from the army and was on the run from the old bill after breaking his wife's boyfriend's legs, as you do. Traumatised by military service, he was well off his trolley and we got on. By complete coincidence it transpired that he'd previously squatted in Camden Road next door to my friend Alan Tyler, who by now was frontman of country-rock stars the Rockingbirds. Initially Alan had woken up one morning, peered from the window of his own squat, and seen a tent pitched in his back garden. *"That's funny"*, Alan had thought, *"I don't remember a tent being in my garden before"*. He went outside to investigate. Andy explained that he was homeless and destitute, and went into detail about his wife's boyfriend's legs. Figuring that this was reasonable, Alan felt reassured and left the retired soldier to get on with reintegrating himself into civilian life from the comfort of the back garden.

After a while, Andy got to know Alan's neighbours and moved into the squat next door – the nature of which was later chronicled in Phil Schoenfelt's cult novel *Junkie Love* – into their airing cupboard. He slept each night in the four-feet square space, his tall, muscular frame hunched into an upright foetal position – replicating exactly how he'd had to sleep back in the trenches in the Falklands, as missiles flew constantly overhead and his comrades and indigenous sheep and penguins were blown to fuck around him. Eventually he moved out, next door to us, but unfortunately soon fell out with a crack dealer living downstairs. Still in possession of firearms from the army, Andy was worried that he might throw a hissy fit and shoot the dealer, and to avoid this he moved for a while back into the airing cupboard before disappearing.

A guy called Pat, newly out of Brixton prison, lived in the flat the other side of Philippa's and began harassing Mina. He refused to believe that I was her boyfriend, and no matter how often she insisted otherwise, chose to convince himself that I was in fact her brother, which was odd considering that I'm a white guy and Mina is of mixed race, her father being from Pakistan. Mina became scared of Pat, so after a year we squatted another flat in a block on the slightly more well-to-do Woodberry Down Estate in Manor House. We gave the keys of the Pembury flat to a homeless friend, Mitch, who after a while was evicted by the council; the last time I looked, a decade or so later, the council still hadn't repaired or let out the place. Pat later resurfaced in my life as a staff member at the Junction, a day ward at the Hackney psychiatric hospital where I later worked.

The amenities weren't too clever in the Pembury flat. The windows were broken though kind of secured with what remained of the steel cages, and during the winter, with no heating, it was fucking freezing. We cooked on a Baby Belling, and there was no hot water. However, we found an old washing machine, which didn't work in the conventional way, but when filled with water it acted as a giant kettle enabling us to have baths, though filling it using a hosepipe system was problematic and flooded the flat downstairs once or twice. The electricity was OK because I'd found the main fuse box in the stairwell. Fortunately, a guy who had lived elsewhere on the block had died shortly before we moved in so I stole his fuses, guessing that he wouldn't need them, and plugged them into our sockets. Life there was austere and poverty-stricken, but it felt all right: for some reason, the happiest periods of my life have tended to coincide with living in squats.

I was studying part-time, commuting to Sussex University to study for an MA in literature and philosophy, taking it rather more seriously than I did as an undergraduate and writing a thesis called *Vagrancy and the Unconscious* which impressed the professors. I was also working part-time as a community development worker for Mind in Tower Hamlets, under the excellent guidance and tutelage of my boss Roz Shaw, from whom I learnt a great deal. I've sometimes been lucky with immediate bosses in workplaces, and many haven't reinforced my natural inclination to rebel against all forms of authority. My role there was to set up a community befriending scheme, staffed by a team of volunteers. Befriending schemes are notoriously difficult to get funding for because their focus is to keep people comparatively well and out of hospital. Most mental health services only seem to attract funding if they deal with people at the most acute stages of their distress, a state of affairs which psychiatric social workers often complain about as they seem to spend all their time rushing around servicing hospitals: dealing with people being sectioned under the mental health act, attending meetings with shrinks and doing pre-discharge paperwork when they'd rather be supporting people in the community to prevent them getting so distressed that hospitalisation becomes seemingly inevitable. Befriending schemes, on the rare occasions where they exist, can help fill the gap. As well as recruiting and supervising volunteers and attaching them to punters who needed empathetic human contact, I'd help the punters out with dealings with the welfare benefits and medical systems, and frequently with problems with the law. For example, a guy named Visvaldis Zilpauss, diagnosed 'schizophrenic' but who from what I could see was disabled primarily by a severe drink problem, kept getting done for drunken driving with or without a licence, and a good word from Mind and the convenient if false excuse that he was mad at the time helped to keep him out of jail. Another punter was a woman whose pen-name was Rosie Logan. She'd gone blind due to complications from diabetes, and had ended up on Rachel ward at the local hospital in Mile End. While inside she decided to write a book about her stay there, and handwrote it on scraps of paper, putting her finger below each completed line then commencing the next line beneath the same finger, so as not to write over the same space and keep it legible. After a few weeks of this she'd accumulated such a pile of A4 sheets that she thought she'd written something of the length of *War and Peace*. In fact, *Rosie in Rachel*, as the book was called when Bloomsbury got round to publishing it, ended up as a slim, attractive and moving hardback. The punters represented a wide cross-section of age, race and gender, and I'd like to think that the scheme gave them quality support and had a subtly beneficial effect.

My boss, Roz Shaw, helped fine-tune my belief that basic common humanity towards the 'mentally ill' was far more efficacious and therapeutic than treating them as 'patients', a word which somehow suggests inferiority but which at least does not try to disguise the power imbalance between themselves and practitioners designated to help them, and is therefore more accurate or at least more honest than 'client' or 'user'. Not 'one of them', at least at this stage, I nevertheless approached them from street level rather than pretending to be from on high, and Roz's wise attitude, energy and compassion were supportive and inspiring in this regard.

This didn't help her with her own bosses. The chair of Mind in Tower Hamlets, Richard Smith, was the public face of a cartel of do-gooders apparently more concerned with promoting their own careers than with genuinely innovative, challenging mental health projects. A day centre, Open House, was the flagship of the firm, and the cartel became determined to relocate resources from other Mind projects – specifically those involving community development, and black and minority ethnic communities – in order to expand the centre's remit and pre-eminence. At one point, the cartel threatened to cut the wages of all staff not directly connected to Open House, to fund pay rises for staff at the centre, a divide and rule tactic. I helped prevent this by undertaking some rabble-rousing and carving up an executive committee meeting, pointing out that we all had legally binding work contracts. However, they managed to use Roz's scatty nature as a pretext to delete her Community Development Manager post, putting her out of a job. My response was to quit mine, deciding that I couldn't work with these people.

I wouldn't claim that all my work in Tower Hamlets was perfect; in fact, part of it revealed my inexperience and naivety. Under-stimulated by running a befriending scheme, which wasn't exactly hard and didn't really tax my brain, I made an exploratory attempt to put into motion the setting up of a user group – THUMP, the acronym for Tower Hamlets Union of Mental Patients. The most vocal 'user' involved with this group was the self-styled 'reverend' Roy Devine who'd stumbled onto the scene. Like many figures in the nascent user movement in those days, he didn't really use mental health services at all; merely pretended to, figuring that the 'mentally ill' were more gullible and easier to manipulate than the leftie and anarchist groups he and others like him had been kicked out of for being a pain in the arse. However, I wasn't aware of this yet.

I was gullible myself. I should have listened to Andy Martin from the Apostles, a former friend of Devine's who'd fallen out with him after he began sending creepy letters and making strange phone calls to Andy's female friends, most notably Lucy Williams, and showing Andy's bassist Dave Fanning his pornography collection. Andy warned me against Devine, and he was right. Before THUMP had even started letting people know it existed, I received a rambling and apparently crazy letter from a woman purporting to be an acquaintance of the fake reverend claiming that he was sexually abusive, and going into graphic detail about carnal activity involving a dog. In our naivety both myself and Roz dismissed the letter as a work of delusion. After I'd stopped operating in Tower Hamlets, THUMP was still holding meetings, and Devine began sending letters to a female group member, purportedly from a fellow user activist John Henderson, threatening to perform perverse and unpleasant acts on this woman, like sticking red hot pokers up her cunt. The threats became so frightening that, apparently, the woman moved house. It transpired that Devine had a long history of sending letters under the names of people he considered his rivals, containing the most foul abuse, threats and slander. At City and Hackney Mind, where Henderson was a management committee member, letters in this vein bearing his name were regularly sent to the committee's chair; it was assumed that Devine was behind them, but the police declined to act citing lack of proof. And he'd had me fooled for a while.

Although the user movement has, to a large extent, got wise and cleaned up its act over the years, there has been a history of ill-intentioned individuals working in bad faith to undermine user groups and the people within them. Usually this is in pursuit of power over people, and involves trying to undermine more talented group members or those seen as figureheads. For example, the following happened after de facto CAPO leader Eric Irwin died, and Frank Bangay – a fine man and great poet – assumed an organisational role with the Campaign Against Psychiatric Oppression, more by default than design. Hugh Lansdowne, a bearded middle-aged man renowned for his suit, tie and briefcase from which he was inseparable, began attending CAPO meetings and took every opportunity to verbally attack Frank and make other group members suspicious of him, hoping to see the poet off and become top dog. In particular Frank's heavy drinking was used against him, with the suggestion that he was somehow unfit to have a prominent role within the group. Eventually the stress resulting from these accusations and the ensuing arguments helped lead Frank to a breakdown and hospital admission, leaving Lansdowne nominally in charge. Without Frank's charisma, integrity and motivational skills, and with members becoming bored with Lansdowne's self-promoting lectures, CAPO quickly fell apart – as, needless to say, did THUMP.

Lansdowne has since been involved with a number of user groups and charities, leaving a trail of destruction in his wake. Aside from undermining people whose popularity and abilities provoked his jealousy, he has demonstrated a routine of getting paid or management committee posts with various groups in South London, primarily Lambeth, and buying thousands of pounds' worth of computer equipment with money the groups haven't had, leaving them bankrupt or nearly so. Such behaviour necessitates a peripatetic lifestyle, as problem 'activists' move their operations from one borough to the next as they're serially sussed out; Devine over the ensuing years was shifting gradually further from central London and was eventually commuting to the suburbs to cause trouble. User group trainspotters also became prominent during the user movement's ascendancy, as essentially harmless characters like Steve Brewer turned up at meetings everywhere a group was set up: it was uncanny how they'd manage to find out about all of them. They'd never contribute any ideas towards practice or debate, but they'd have an encyclopaedic knowledge of which activist was in which group, which groups and individuals had been in dispute with each other, and when. If ever a comprehensive history of the user movement is to be written, Brewer would be able to provide great source material concerning the family tree of its personnel.

Mina and I were ensconced in our new squatted studio flat in Manor House. Though small, it had hot running water, central heating, electricity, intact double-glazed windows, the works! And we didn't have to spend a penny on rent or bills! This was the life and it was a happy time. In 1992, after a year there, Mina decided that we should get a mortgage and so we bought a two bedroom flat in Philip Lane, Tottenham, for the then market price of forty grand. We were going up in the world and joining the landed gentry!

We gave the Woodberry Down flat keys to my friend Ewan Murray, who was escaping from the perpetual madness of Andy Martin's house in London Fields. He lived there for a few weeks before waking one morning to find that a small red stain had appeared from nowhere on the ceiling overnight. As the day wore on, the stain enlarged, until after a while red drops began dripping to the floor. Ewan investigated: it was blood!

Worried, he called the emergency services. It transpired that an elderly Polish recluse in the flat above had fallen, dead, hitting his head in the process and spilling what seemed like gallons of blood. The old guy had lived there for over a decade. Nobody knew him. In one of the most densely populated areas of Western Europe, it's all too easy to be unnoticed and alone.

Traumatised, Ewan moved out, and John, Philippa's ex-partner and father of her baby Callum, moved in. After a few weeks, John came back from his habitual day's ducking and diving to find the flat secured with a steel door and steel windows and with some of his possessions piled outside, the rest locked inside. When he levered the door off to retrieve his stuff, a high-pitched whistle screeched out at ear-splitting volume audible from miles away. He located the offending alarm and threw it from the window, leaving it still whistling on the grass between two blocks, two stories below. The next-door neighbours threatened to kill John, being as they were on the illiberal side. Not realising we were squatters, they'd been pleased when Mina and myself had moved in as the previous occupants had been "*disgusting lesbians*" and therefore likely to spread diseases and fiddle with the local kids. Not that the local kids needed corrupting: the girls growing up on the estate were, without exception, pushing prams around by the age of sixteen whilst the boys amused themselves with gang-brawls and breaking open the washing machines in the nearby launderette in broad daylight in front of the customers, in vain attempts to liberate the coins inside. I didn't care. I was completing my MA, settling into my new flat and preparing for my new job – advocacy co-ordinator with City and Hackney Mind.

Shake Some Action

Half an hour before my interview for the Advocacy Co-ordinator post at City and Hackney Mind, I went to Andy Martin's place in London Fields and shared a spliff with Apostles bassist Dave Fanning. It was far stronger than I'd anticipated, and I arrived at the interview grinning like an idiot. Roger Harris, then director of the show, led me upstairs into the interview room when it was my turn.

Mental health advocacy was a new phenomenon at the time, and the project I set up in Hackney was one of the first of its kind in Britain. At the interview I was met by a couple of female voluntary sector workers from specific minority ethnic communities; David Ndegwa, a black forensic psychiatrist, and Roger, a white guy who'd tried to be politically correct by making the panel diverse. Maybe I said the right things, but I think it more likely that it was my stoned, comforting demeanour got me the job, endearing the panel to me. I wondered what on earth the other people they'd interviewed must have been like, although Roger assured me later that there had been a strong field.

Safely holed up in Tottenham and fit enough at the time to charge into work every day on my bicycle, I set up the project very quickly. There were very few advocacy services at the time to copy, but Mind in Tower Hamlets had some paperwork including policies and procedures, and I ripped some of these off, changing the odd word here and there and also slipping in some more radical stuff from groups in Holland and of all places, Nottingham, both of which were atypically advanced in terms of acknowledging and asserting psychiatric patients' rights. Advocacy projects at the time were meant to protect patients' rights by allowing them to have people with and acting for them to help articulate their interests – as they perceived them – in situations affecting their treatment and welfare: for example interviews with psychiatrists, nurses and social workers, and dealings with housing and welfare benefits agencies. This required advocates to be fully conversant with the Mental Health Act 1983 and other laws, as well as to be lucid and articulate. For some years, mental health service user groups had been demanding the setting up of advocacy services in the mental health field, aware that, particularly in hospitals, rights were routinely abused, and the concept of advocacy was perceived by advocates and professionals alike to have an oppositional content which some professionals felt threatened by, even though advocates had no powers enshrined in law. Advocacy services have flourished and become embedded in the mental health system over the years since, at the cost of being co-opted and losing their oppositional status. The project was up and running within a few weeks and I soon met my first 'clients'.

The first was a woman named Avril Ali, who had been discharged from Strauss Ward at St. Batholomews Hospital in the City of London, which was within the advocacy project's catchment area. She arrived home from hospital to discover that one of the nurses, who'd blagged her house-keys from her thinking that she'd be incarcerated for longer than she eventually was, had installed into her flat in Hackney a relative of his who had recently migrated unofficially into the country from Uganda. Bizarrely, Avril and the Ugandan chick lived in the flat together for a while, the latter feeling too confused about the situation to leave of her own accord and perhaps unaware that there was anything strange about the set-up, with Avril not assertive enough to challenge her. The nurse kept his distance from the situation. After talking to Avril I brought the issue to light at her request and the nurse's relative was forced to move somewhere else. I felt sorry for the Ugandan woman, but also felt that the nurse's behaviour had been abusive, as well as plain crazy. Astonishingly, the nurse kept his job on the grounds that it was a first offence and out of character. I don't know what became of his cousin.

Avril, who had unfeasibly long curly fingernails and seemed easily manipulated, continued over the years to have a succession of problematic characters using her flat, mostly crack dealers, and she never went on to think of the place solely as hers.

On my first day at work, I was shown around PICU: the dreaded psychiatric intensive care unit, the lock-up ward at the Hackney Hospital where in theory the eighteen most acutely psychotic people in the borough at any one time were incarcerated. There was a high ratio of nurses to patients, and any loud behaviour or perceived misdemeanour by the patients would lead to them being 'restrained' by half a dozen nurses and injected with Largactyl. The prospect of being sent there was issued as a threat to patients on the other, less intensive wards who were seen as non-compliant. Each patient on PICU was given a daily cocktail of enough anti-psychotic drugs to knock out an entire family. When I arrived there were seventeen young black men, and one white woman who approached me and offered me sweets: Debbie McNamara.

A few weeks later Debbie – sane, lucid and highly intelligent – visited my office asking for help to complain about the way in which she'd been admitted to that ward, which she felt had involved a series of misunderstandings. We got on and became friends, as to a lesser extent I did with some of the black guys on the ward: when I've been threatened on Hackney's streets since, on more than one occasion someone I've known from PICU, or indeed other wards, has stepped in and said *"leave that bloke alone, he's all right!"* My work in the bin has indirectly helped prevent me from being mugged, and smoothed over a variety of other potentially hazardous situations.

Owing to the fact that back then there were very few templates to follow when setting up advocacy projects, I started a North East London Advocacy Network to share ideas and problems with other workers developing similar services, so that we could essentially make it all up as we went along. Gradually over the years this would mutate into the much larger Greater London Advocacy Network, led primarily by a suit in superficially informal clothes named Jonathan Coe, who went on to campaign for advocacy 'standards' and mandatory professional qualifications without which advocates would become unable to practice. Interventions such as his would, over the years, lead to mental health advocacy becoming, much of the time, simply another professional tier like nursing or social work, with psychiatric patients requiring peer advocates to approach and negotiate with their professional advocates. This situation would coincide with advocacy being taken more seriously within the system, at a great price. But in 1992 everything was up for grabs.

An advocate – as envisaged from the user movement's perspective – was a comrade helping you to communicate with professionals, as well as fulfilling administrative tasks which you might have trouble doing by yourself, either because of incapacity through distress or lack of access to information. It's a task best undertaken by other people who have been through the system as users themselves, people with their own problems who can understand and speak with you on your own level, cutting through all the jargon and bullshit, unlike many community psychiatric nurses and social workers who – skilled and well-intentioned though they uasually are – cannot communicate on an equal footing simply because of the amount of power they have. An advocate cannot section you under the mental health act or arrange for your kids to go into care; but if advocates become official professionals then there is a risk that they would begin to identify and collude with those workers who patients may perceive to be on the other side. Over time, there has indeed been a drift in this direction. Real advocates should refuse to eat in staff canteens, be cognisant with street slang and dress with their arse hanging out of their trousers. But people like Coe have helped make mental health advocacy more bureaucratic and professional, rendering it meaningless.

I recruited a string of advocates, some of them volunteers, others paid, the first of the latter being the African Caribbean advocate Sasere Obaseki. She was pretty efficient, though not passionately committed to the cause of mental patients' rights in the way that I had become. For her it was simply a job, which was fair enough, but this occasionally led to friction and sometimes she seemed exasperated by my lax and not strictly boundaried approach to the work. On one occasion, I had to challenge her for being homophobic. In front of me and my friend Phil Murphy – and for all she knew either of us could have been gay or bisexual – she announced: *"Well, of course, we'd all prefer people to be heterosexual – being gay just isn't natural"*. Actually Phil and I are straight but that was hardly the point, so I at once told her to keep her opinions to herself.

"What you're saying is racist!" she claimed. *"In the black community, nobody likes homosexuals! And in the land of my heritage, Nigeria, there's no such thing as homosexuality anyway! All gays are white people!"*

Jesus Christ, I thought to myself, before laying down the law: a rare occasion when I've felt obliged to seriously have a go at someone whose boss I've been. She shut up. But inadvertently she'd raised some kind of an issue. In Tottenham where I lived, posters appeared constantly on walls, at bus stops, even on the inside of shop windows advertising the so-called Marcus Garvey History Club, which presented itself as a discussion group debating topics such as *"Women – why their place is in the home"*, *"Batty boys – why we should eliminate them"* and *"The protocols of the elders of Zion – true or false?"* These wankers supposed themselves to be black nationalists, and were a mirror image – some might say a photographic negative – of the British National Party. They helped to indicate that nationalism is, by definition, a form of fascism.

During my stint at the advocacy project, we developed a high profile and a reputation for being committed and effective, making it very difficult for hospital staff to abuse their patients without being called to account, although sadly this situation receded over the years after I left the job. On the occasions when I came onto a professional's case if I thought they were dodgy, I'd spy on them for as long as I needed to until they slipped up and I managed to nail them. Staff had a habit of closing ranks and protecting their own even in the most outrageous situations, but usually incontrovertible proof of professional misconduct would arise sooner or later. Unfortunately some very nasty people did get away with it. For example, in 1999 the ward manager of PICU, a biker named Dennis Drake, took it upon himself to physically 'restrain' a psychotic, eight months pregnant woman by sitting on her stomach. The staff all claimed that this incident simply hadn't taken place, scared of Drake and the ward psychiatrist Jim Lucey, who I suspected may have routinely colluded with abuses and cover-ups including this one. The entire staff claimed that all eighteen patients on the ward had experienced a mysterious collective delusion in an example of occult mass hysteria. I didn't witness the incident, and it was one demographic group's word against another's, but I know who I believed. When I raised the issue in front of his boss, Drake threatened to sue me for slander.

Nobody was called to account for this specific incident, but Dr Jim Lucey was caught out in the end for something else. At the time, psychiatric hospitals were required to have a statutory board of 'hospital managers', basically unpaid laymen who traditionally convened from time to time to rubber-stamp issues of hospital practice, procedure and use of the Mental Health Act. With the introduction of advocacy, patients' rights were starting to be asserted in hospitals in subtle ways, and with the help of the hospital Mental Health Act administrator Gloria Brown who was sympathetic to our cause, more questioning individuals began to appear within the board of managers. Hospital Managers' hearings had the power to discharge patients from sections against the doctors' advice, although prior to the rise of advocacy services this power was never used, and certainly not at the Hackney Hospital. In the case of Ray Brown, who seemed perfectly fine to me but whom Lucey was threatening with gratuitous forensic examinations, apparently trying to fast-track the patient to Broadmoor for no apparent reason, the managers were happy to let him go. Lucey, his power threatened and feeling the size of his dick diminish inside his trousers, wasn't having it and informed the nursing staff that Brown was in fact still detained under a section. When the patient went back to the ward to collect his stuff, he was set upon by nurses who refused to let him go.

"If Dr Lucey told you to rob a bank, would you go and do it?" I used the old cliché to confront the nurses with the following morning. They were afraid to disobey the eminent consultant psychiatrist even if it meant compromising themselves by breaking the law. I don't know what they thought would happen to them if they did: perhaps his clinical gaze would melt them into a puddle of molten haloperidol on the floor of the ward? Even Lisa Cunningham, the so-called rock'n'roll nurse we'd named after the character in the New York Dolls' version of the old Bo Diddley standard *Pills*, kept quiet and stared at her shoes along with the rest of them. None of them had the guts to stand up to the rogue doctor.

During the night of his illegal incarceration, Brown complained to the staff about not being allowed to leave. As a punishment for this he was held down by six nurses who forcibly injected him with tranquillising anti-psychotic drugs in the arse. I was back on the case the next day, clarified Ray's legal situation for him, and got hold of a decent solicitor and the local rag the

Hackney Gazette. The management in charge of the hospital, the paid variety this time, became very nervous as awkward questions were put to them. It turned out that the local mental health trust had to come up with a five figure sum in damages and legal fees for false imprisonment and assault to prevent the case from going to court and the bad publicity that would have ensued: buying silence. Lucey, literally in tears, quietly resigned from his post, his manhood in tatters, and he got a job as a lecturer at St Bartholomews Hospital where he could keep a lower profile and do less damage.

Some of the other psychiatrists were also pretty weird. A case in point was Dr Jeremy Coyde, an old-school shrink who was jointly in charge of the interim secure unit, a forensic ward which was essentially an outpost of Broadmoor. It accommodated offenders with enduring mental health issues and criminal records, and some of the guys there had done terrible things. Others – particularly the black guys – had simply drifted into the place following dubious, gratuitous forensic assessments whose findings portended potential dangers in the future. Coyde's co-consultant, Dr David Ndegwa, was a personable, charming and seemingly highly-principled practitioner who became well-respected for advancing the cause of multicultural awareness within his field, writing books on the subject; how he managed to work with Coyde remains a mystery. Coyde claimed to have invented some 'treatment' techniques for people with 'severe personality disorders' hitherto deemed as untouchable, but his demeanour mirrored that of the most unemotional of the people he was trying to control. Nicknamed 'Android Coyde' by the patients owing to his complete lack of discernible human emotions, empathy or warmth, he gave me the fucking creeps. Once I was at a mental health review tribunal with a black man who, 23 years previously at the age of 15, had been hospitalised for stealing a pair of curtains from a church he'd slept in whilst homeless. The patient had, over time, drifted ever further into the forensic mental health system, due to behaviour such as altercations with staff who were attempting to give him forced injections of psychiatric medication that he didn't want. Coyde wanted to send him to Broadmoor and throw away the key. I pointed out to the tribunal that the patient may have been led to his current situation by incremental institutional racism within the mental health care system, an allegation which appalled the robotic, scientific

Android in attendance. If Coyde's looks could kill I would have dropped dead there and then. My client blew it by stating that he thought he'd been sentenced in the first place only because the judge had been jealous that he was the one and only son of God, and he was duly sent to Broadmoor on the doctor's recommendation. If he's still alive, he probably remains there. Coyde's clinical gaze was always chilling, like something out of a horror film. I was once in a lift with him. I was scared out of my wits. *"I can smell alcohol"*, he told me, *"have you taken a drink?"* I denied it, and I was being truthful, as his cold and hateful glare sent evil shivers down my spine.

Some of my thinking then remained naïve. I used to challenge people using the term 'mental illness' and other medical terminology, to the extent that I unsuccessfully lobbied for a swear box to be put in the office so that I could make people stick coins into it whenever they were caught using the offending words. But while the term 'mental illness' presupposes the dominance of the medical model in comprehending human distress and has no scientific basis, it nevertheless makes sense as a metaphor. For example, from bitter experience I am aware that real physical symptoms arise from depression, which may or may not include insomnia, appetite loss or gain, sexual dysfunction, fatigue and a whole list of others in addition to whatever is going on in your mind. You certainly don't feel very well.

Among the advocates I recruited there was a succession of Turkish workers. Hackney's refugee and asylum seeker population was predominantly Turkish and Kurdish, and these communities were well accounted for in the hospital: nearly all of the patients unable to speak English were able to speak Turkish. The workers included Sozen Ismail, Zehra Ocal, Sevim Clegg and Tuba Karacalar, all women. As well as these, volunteers over the five years during which I ran the project included Terry Conway, Leila Salim, Dan McQuillan, Andrea Lambert, Jo Crane, Debbie McNamara, Ruth Roberts, Phil Murphy, Earil Hunter, Ralph Gibbons and many others.

The advocacy project was at first installed into a disused room in the basement beneath F-block, the building which accommodated most of the wards. It had broken windows, no amenities and the threadbare carpets were infested with mould. Plaster was peeling from the walls and lumps of concrete fell randomly at regular intervals from the ceiling. A permanent waft of canna-

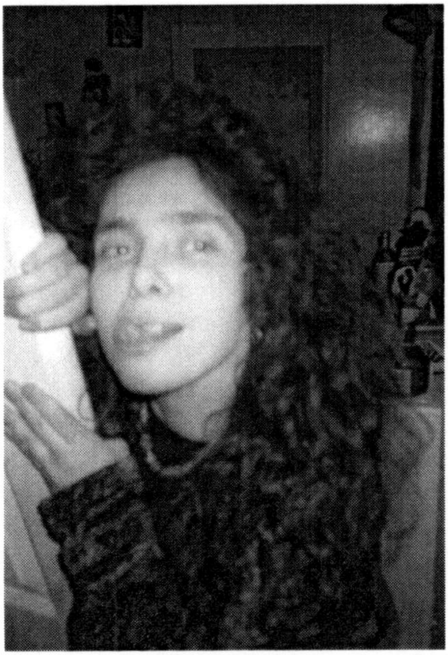
Sozen Ismail

bis generally helped obscure the odour of brick dust, neighbouring blocks being in the process of demolition, and also that of sewage, the plumbing being past its sell by date at the old Hackney hospital. Vomit and disinfectant also featured heavily, because the smell of these permeates all hospitals. I'd given up smoking fags whilst in Croydon after having a panic attack for the first time, involving hyperventilation and overdosing on oxygen, accelerating heartbeat like a drum machine speeding into a high-pitched whirr, out of control anxiety, fainting: the works. At the time I wasn't aware what a panic attack was, and thought I might be having a heart attack. This encouraged me to quit, but soon after I kidded myself that cannabis sprinkled into tobacco in spliffs wasn't really smoking. I re-addicted myself to nicotine, and before long I was smoking joints with alarming regularity. My boss Roger made one or two subtle comments about the smell of it in the office but chose not to pursue the matter. Meanwhile, alien varieties of mushrooms sprouted in large clusters from all corners of the room and glutinous green slime regularly oozed through the walls and covered the carpets emitting acrid smoke. I felt perfectly at home.

Sozen wandered into this dilapidated office wearing a large overcoat which was quivering manically, apparently of its own accord. *"What's wrong with your coat?"* I asked her.

"It's my pigeon!" she explained, unbuttoning her coat and reaching inside. She removed the young bird from her clothing and plonked it onto the desk in front of her. The desk collapsed, one of its legs deciding to break, not being able to take the extra weight, and drawers shot out spilling their contents. *"I found it in the gutter in Homerton High Street"*, she continued, *"and the poor*

thing's ill". It was. It couldn't spread its wings, it made asthmatic noises and it had a runny beak. It was well off colour and generally looked sorry for itself. Perhaps it had been abandoned too soon by its mother. I got the desk working again by replacing the broken leg with a pile of old medical records I'd found outside. The young pigeon looked as if it was about to throw up. Sozen took the pigeon back with her back to her flat, which was already home to 25 cats she'd found astray around her estate, the Kingsmead. Isolating the bird in her bathroom, she fed and nurtured it with homeopathic treatments, herbal remedies and cat food until eventually it got better and flew away.

Zehra, Tuba, Sevim and Sozen were all competent advocates trying to do a very hard job, dealing with punters marginalised not only by being carted off to a psychiatric hospital – usually against their will – engendering extreme stigma and prejudice from within their own communities, but who also couldn't even speak the same language as the doctors and nurses who were supposed to be treating them. There was no effective interpreting service in the hospital. The advocacy service filled some of the gaps: it wasn't strictly our role to provide interpreting, but this was necessary simply to enable any advocacy to take place at all with this group, and none of us could bear to see these doubly disempowered punters abandoned any more than they already were. Eventually we gained sufficient evidence of the plight of, and lack of support for Turkish and Kurdish patients to convince City and East London Health Authority to give us money for a permanent Turkish advocate post for four days a week. Zehra Ocal's sister Hatice got the job, and she worked very long hours above and beyond what she was paid for, buzzing around the bin like a blue-arsed fly interpreting, liaising with solicitors, doctors, nurses, social workers, benefits officers, cops, all manner of bureaucrats and authority figures, trying to make life half-way bearable for a gang of extremely distressed Turks and Kurds. If Hatice and the other workers hadn't been there, their clients would have been fucked and some of them probably would have topped themselves.

Some of the Turkish clients presented the most difficult and heartbreaking cases the project dealt with. One Kurd, Hassan Hassan had, he told me, been a simple sheep-farmer's son in the mountains of Eastern Turkey, following his father's occupational footsteps. The PKK, a Kurdish liberation outfit loathed by the

Turkish government, established an armed guerrilla base there in the mountains. Hassan was tending his sheep one morning when the PKK came across him and gave him a thorough interrogation. Realising he was harmless to them, they let him go, warning him to keep his mouth shut to the authorities about their presence but confiscating his address book which contained his personal details.

Shortly after this, the official Turkish military forces attacked the PKK's mountain base, killing all of the guerrillas. The army found the address book and passed it to the local cops who took Hassan in for questioning, figuring he was somehow connected to the liberation fighters. Hassan was tortured very badly in the police cells and had his testicles removed, and he was threatened with far worse unless they gave him information he didn't have. Somehow he managed to escape and he fled to England.

When he arrived, he faced the full force of the British system's disrespect and insensitivity towards those fleeing danger and persecution in foreign lands. Hassan was separated from his family and everyone and everything he had ever known. He was baffled by a strange culture, unable to speak a word of English, could not communicate with any officialdom, and became an asylum seeker, not really knowing what that meant or entailed. He had no money, no food or accommodation to speak of, and a complicated court case ahead of him. Not surprisingly, he wound up in hospital severely depressed after a suicide attempt. Some people object to what they consider the liberal treatment of refugees and asylum seekers in this country. If they knew how desperate many of these people are: what they have tried to escape, and how, and all of the horrors involved, these objectors would alter their opinions if they have any kind of heart.

Hassan encountered the indignity of working with an immigration solicitor who made no attempt whatsoever to discover the asylum seeker's true history or any of the details relevant to his application. The lawyer didn't even bother locating an interpreter: he just knew that he could make some money out of the legal aid system. It took Tuba Karacalar a long time to gain Hassan's trust and get the whole picture from him during his stay in hospital. Armed with information, we found him a less cynical lawyer and we negotiated with the relevant authorities to get him welfare benefits, along with support from torture victim charities and social workers able to work with people who don't speak

English, and a place to live of sorts. But even after his discharge from hospital he'd still come back to the advocacy office every day for a year or so, telling us that our little room was the only place in London where he felt safe. His depression persisted. At his squat, another Turkish guy threatened to stab him because of a minor dispute. *"Go on then"* Hassan said to the knife-wielding aggressor, *"I want to die anyway"*. The other resident didn't oblige. I hope Hassan is okay now.

Dan McQuillan, meanwhile, was a frighteningly clever man who had a PhD in physics and was as hard as fuck. Honestly, you'd really want this guy on your side if there was a ruck. Trained in martial arts and armed with brutal, quick-witted cunning, he was our secret weapon.

Such skills weren't strictly necessary for him to befriend and attempt to advocate for patients on Joshua ward, a long-term, locked rehabilitation unit for severely institutionalised and dependent people. The ward was heartbreaking: the turnover of patients was dismally slow, and with few exceptions the same fifteen people were kept under lock and key in a small space for year after year, without having committed any 'crime' save unremitting painful psychosis. Every one of these patients was doped with complex combinations of psychotropic drugs in quantities far beyond the recommended limits, with dubious legality. The drugs had no effect in reducing these patients' psychosis, and merely made them quieter and more docile: in fact, they were fast asleep for most of the time. One patient, Rachel Gerber, spoke six or seven languages and flitted between them incomprehensibly in a verbal confusion. She had no idea at all where she was, or even who she was, but usually believed that her husband – who had divorced her twenty years earlier – was due to collect her any day and take her home. Occasionally, a crack would appear in her psychotic armour and an inkling of insight into the unending horror of her situation would creep in. The terrible reality would be too much for her to take, and she'd escape by retreating even further into her jumbled world of delusion. If she's still alive she's probably still on a rehab unit now. This was the dreaded Joshua Ward, and Dan and Terry Conway nobly and patiently got to know the folks there, trying to use any available avenue to get them out of the place: anywhere would have been better. This was easier said than done, and any sensitive person visiting Joshua Ward would emerge heartbroken and angry.

Dan, an anarchist, liked to channel his anger by rucking the old bill. I wouldn't wish to be a copper when Dr McQuillan's around; I'd be looking at several months in hospital. In 2001, the anarcho-scientist went to Genoa to protest against a G5 summit, which was a mass-meeting of the cunts who rule the world. During the protests, Dan was asleep on the floor in an old school which was temporarily being used as an independent media centre, along with dozens of other anti-globalisation protesters. That night, the carabinieri broke into the school. There are two police forces in Italy: the polizia, relatively speaking the friendly bobbies on the beat, and the real hard bastards the carabinieri, a militia renowned for violence, racism, and close connections with shadowy neo-fascist movements and mafia-style criminal gangs. These goons kicked fuck out of Dan and his mates while they were asleep. If Dan had been awake, he'd have taken on the whole lot of them and probably won. In the event he became a media celebrity, pictured on the front covers of most of Britain's daily newspapers with his shiner, cuts and bruises and broken arm in a sling, alongside the other four English protesters who'd been arrested and beaten up, one of whom was Norman Blair, former editor of *Class War.* Dan and his comrades were tortured in an Italian cop shop before being deported, and the Italian state was given a suitably hard time in the media for laying into these peaceful, gentle extremists who wouldn't hurt a fly. We were very fortunate to have a man of Dan's calibre onside at the advocacy project, and he was popular and well-respected among patients and staff alike, as was Terry, whose account of his prodigious use of hallucinogenic drugs leading to breakdown and hospitalisation in the 1960s is documented hilariously and in his own words in the classic anthology *Mad Pride: A Celebration of Mad Culture* (Spare Change, 2000). In denial about his mad status for many years for fear of stigma and rejection from his working-class peers, Terry chose to make sense of and reclaim his experience by working for us, and as it turned out his mates' respect for him remained intact when he 'came out' as a former psychiatric patient. A skilled, committed and compassionate man who'd help anyone, he went on to become chair of the Hackney Patients Council, and eventually a psychiatric social worker, one of the best.

I was so lucky to amass such a brave, intelligent and good-hearted crew around me. It was hard work for all of us. At least I was being paid: the volunteers were there solely out of altruism. Andrea Lambert for example was an extremely efficient volunteer advocate who was there virtually full time, prolifically getting results; I was never quite sure exactly what her background was, but she treated staff and patients alike as equals, whereas more gullible people working in hospitals would have looked up to paid workers, especially those in senior positions, and down on the patients. She took on Sasere's African Caribbean advocate post as a locum when Sasere took maternity leave, and shortly afterwards landed a permanent mental health advocacy job at the Whittington hospital in Archway, which was our loss and their gain. Ruth Roberts, still grieving for her husband who'd recently died young, also pulled her weight before ending up on remand in Holloway women's prison on a fraud charge; they let her go after a trial. I still see her in the street from time to time: she tries to persuade me to embrace the Lord and attend her local church. I'd met Ralph, Jo and Debbie when they were patients at the hospital who wished to give something back, or else take revenge. Ralph, a depressed, elderly gay guy, was particularly effective with his painstaking work with long term, institutionalised rehab patients.

Part of the deal with this project was that we encountered the same old problems again and again as we dealt with clients on an individual basis. Many doctors wouldn't listen to their patients' own perspectives on their experiences: they didn't believe the user movement slogan that 'we are the experts on our own distress'. Overstretched social workers, unable to perform the preventative community support work most of them wished to, were under pressure solely to service the hospital, spending all their time performing statutory work around admissions and discharges until the revolving door swung around again. The welfare benefits system in Hackney was a complete shambles, and at one point less than half of the people in the borough who had applied and were eligible for housing benefit were actually getting any due to the system's complexity and the borough's failure to process the applications. People were on social housing waiting lists for decades while thousands of council properties remained derelict for year after year. There was coercion, stigma, nurses unable to speak out against malpractice for justified fear of adversely affecting their careers; and the Hackney hospital was falling to bits. Life was hard for Hackney's psychiatric patients.

The Hackney hospital was located in Homerton, one of the most deprived parts of Western Europe and rough even by Hackney standards. Over the years Homerton had become a psychiatric ghetto. Most of the borough's inpatient and community mental health services came to be based there, alongside drug clinics, residential units and the notorious sink estate, the Kingsmead. A walk along Homerton High Street would take you past very few pedestrians who hadn't used mental health services, though the district's reputation as a dustbin for nutters wasn't new but had a long history.

Hackney Poor House opened its doors in the High Street in 1729, housing fifteen local paupers. It moved across the road in 1741 to a bigger building where there were thirty paupers. By 1764 the number of paupers had been increased to 48, spread across a total of five rooms. Various huts and sheds were annexed; by 1834 the already high local level of deprivation had been worsened by epidemics of cholera and smallpox, and no fewer than 380 of Hackney's poor lived in the complex. It goes without saying that many of these residents were mad.

After 1841 the institution was revamped and new buildings were erected, buildings which were inhabited right up until Hackney hospital's eventual closure in 1995. The new set-up was a Victorian workhouse with as many as 1,030 inmates by 1930, plus an additional 663 people who were medically monitored in the workhouse infirmary. From 1930, the institution stopped being a workhouse and was reclassified as a hospital, in the same way that many psychiatric units in Europe mutated, tellingly, out of leper colonies during the middle ages. At first it housed a wide range of medical disciplines, but by the time the advocacy project arrived the place was being run down. Many of the buildings had already been abandoned; the only inmates left were mad ones.

The first two years of my five and a half year stint as advocacy co-ordinator were spent in this dump, the past echoing through the ages into the present. It was as if the whole place was haunted. Building and demolition were taking place, in part preparing for the erection of a new medium-secure unit, on the site which would be a kind of localised mini-Broadmoor, the Health Authority figuring that it would be cheaper to house patients from the borough on forensic sections locally rather than in private institutions or the famous special hospitals. The non-forensic psychiatric wards were earmarked for removal to a brand new building on the site of the Homerton general hospital around the corner. The building works, often combined with the oppressive heat from the hospital central heating system which had two settings – off, and on full blast – and mixed in too with the sewage which regularly engulfed the lower floors of F-block, made the place an unhealthy environment to work in, let alone be a patient for years on end. In common with many others I developed severe facial rashes during this time, something I've suffered from neither before nor since.

Helping patients get their welfare benefits, though not technically our job, became a heavy demand on the advocacy service, due entirely to the scarcity of other agencies offering this kind of support. We did our best, with our backs to the wall. Local social workers and CPNs were overworked and overwhelmed, as also were we, and in any case they frequently weren't skilled enough to get their heads around the welfare benefits system well enough to be of much use to their clients. There was a hospital 'benefits worker', Bob Lepper. However, he seemed primarily concerned with grassing people up to the dole if they'd been in hospital for six weeks or more, after which inpatients' benefits were immediately and greatly decreased by law. Lepper saw himself as the hospital benefits gatekeeper, apparently believing that patients didn't deserve any more than the pittance to which they were technically entitled, which wouldn't even have kept an ordinary person in tobacco for more than three days in a week let along pay for extras. Lepper never seemed to consider that the hard graft involved with helping people to maximise their benefits might turn out to be as rewarding a power trip as plunging patients into poverty.

The doctors and nurses, with the odd rare exception, weren't trying to make their patients' lives worse, but they were toiling within an oppressive and irrational regime giving too much credence to the medical model, which in turn was and is over-dependent on the pharmaceutical industry and its pathological striving for pathologising, and by turn, profiting, generally at the expense of those on whom it pushes its products. While I don't hold that psychiatric drugs never have any good use, I find it difficult to trust products marketed for the sole reason of making money at all costs, and whose circulation has frequently been dependent on research results falsified by their manufacturers. If psychiatric drugs were that effective and didn't have terribly debilitating side effects, the pharmaceutical complex wouldn't need laws coercing people to take the drugs against their will, and wouldn't be paying agencies to lobby for changes in the law increasing the range of people who can be coerced. This industry is widely considered to be among the most lucrative and corrupt corporate business sector in the world. Up to and during my early days at the Hackney hospital, I would tend to blame the psychiatric profession for the abuses it inflicts upon those it purports to help. Over time I modified this belief and saw the wider picture, realising that the essential problem is capitalism. Psychiatry is compromised by the fact that it has willingly been manoeuvred into a position of dominance in the field of treating and containing human misery, as a servant of profit and social control. Some psychiatrists are even beginning to suspect as much themselves.

Given these systemic problems it seems reasonable to me that pressure groups should exist to challenge them in systemic ways. A group was needed at the Hackney hospital to bring to light and challenge common failures, informed by the recurring individual problems and abuses tackled repetitively by the advocacy service.

Gary Gilmore's Eyes

In 1994, my friend Phil Murphy relocated from Brighton to London to escape the attentions of a violent psychopath who'd been on his case on the south coast. At a loose end, he volunteered for the advocacy service, but found the face to face, one-to-one work a grind. Meanwhile, a charismatic revolving-door patient, Earil Hunter, was a former member of the British karate team. If he'd had a fight with Dan McQuillan, it would have been hard to predict the winner. Black, strong and standing at six feet five, the nurses felt intimidated by him, giving him more restrictive and coercive treatment than would have been the case if he'd been small and white. If he was unconscious much of the time because of enormous quantities of super-strength antipsychotic drugs, he'd be perceived as less of a threat. I liked him, admiring his wit and intelligence, which persisted throughout his ordeals in hospital. I was inspired by some previous work I'd undertaken on a sessional basis with Mina Sassoon, Pete Fleischmann and others for the charity Good Practices In Mental Health: it had been a survey of current patients' opinions of their treatment and the conditions in north-west London hospitals under the Parkside health authority's auspices, involving guided interviews and statistical analysis resulting in a report, which Parkside had commissioned but buried for their own protection when they saw what it was like. I decided to organise a similar survey at Hackney hospital and got Phil and Earil to conduct the interviews using questionnaires we'd designed.

At most hospitals, which are better managed and where a closer eye is kept on what goes on, such an undertaking would be unthinkable. Its concept and methodology would have to be run past an ethics committee, existing by statute, and there would be all manner of other hurdles and interrogation. In Hackney nobody seemed to have heard of the idea of ethics committees and therefore there simply wasn't one. Our methods were hardly scientific but resulted, I think, in an accurate snapshot of what the hospital was like.

Jo Crane was working for Gallup as a qualified social researcher, and gave us some advice which lent us a vestige of credibility. Phil and Earil floated around the bin unchallenged for a few weeks, conducting guided interviews about a comprehensive range of hospital-related issues; treatment, social conditions leading to admission, diet on the wards, safety, anything and everything else we could think of. The hospital food, incidentally, was delivered to the wards on metal trolleys known by most as 'muck trucks', and I wonder what results would have surfaced if somebody had surveyed patients' vitamin deficiencies and long-term illnesses caused by poor nutrition, the food consisting of sludgy over-boiled vegetables followed by pink blancmange; the medication, meanwhile, was delivered on a 'jolly trolley'. The nurses were especially pissed off with Earil's involvement, worrying that he'd have an axe to grind. In fact he and Phil conducted the interviews assiduously and conscientiously, without putting words into the patients' mouths.

After the interviews had been statistically analysed and presented in a pseudo-meaningful way by Phil, Earil and myself, a book was printed, blandly entitled *A Report Concerning Conditions at the Hackney Hospital as Seen By The Patients*. Copies of the book were sent to local and national papers and magazines, together with a press release signposting the more controversial aspects of the book's contents. The result was devastating, possibly putting the final nail into the hospital's coffin and preventing any possibility of the institution's last-minute reprieve.

"Hospital of Horror Slammed in Report", read the front-page headline of the *Tower Hamlets Gazette*. The article was neatly juxtaposed beside a photograph of a 17-year-old girl with huge tits who'd won a local beauty contest. Among quotes selected by

the paper was a patient's comment about the wards' cleanliness which we'd listed as 'positive' feedback: *"Yes, the toilets are clean, because I personally clean them out"*. On women's safety: *"it's naughty, I get up to no good"*. The paper had selected all the quotes that its readers could be shocked or titillated by. Hospital staff were livid, and as equally uncomplimentary pieces appeared in the *Hackney Gazette, Nursing Times, Community Care, Health Services Journal* and others, a scandal grew. I was scared to go to work at the hospital for a while during this media explosion. I was worried that I'd be beaten up by some of the more aggressive nurses before being kicked off the site and told never to return. If Dan and Earil hadn't been around I'd probably never have gone near the place again. By then, the advocacy service had moved into another, larger room, ironically an old ECT suite which still had a disused ECT machine lurking eerily in the corner, which we perversely kept there as a mascot. But although I received numerous hostile stares and funny looks, I wasn't seriously challenged; in fact, the staff began to regard me with a combination of fear and awe. With the other advocacy workers, I'd proved the seriousness of my intent, and suddenly we had the run of the place with the staff too scared to challenge us, and so we looked for the opportunities to exploit this fact.

The next step was to set up Hackney Patients Council, which I envisaged as a union of inpatients fighting for improved conditions and rights for themselves. This project eventually went wrong, but for a short while it breathed fresh air, humanity and real life into a dump which, in its various guises, had traditionally been run in an authoritarian way from the top down over the centuries.

The shadowy conspirators administering the hospital site with their panoptic gaze were now finding things a struggle: their observation systems were falling to bits around them along with the institution generally, which was gradually closing down and becoming abandoned. Undemolished areas of the site were too numerous and far-flung to be policed twenty-four seven by the hospital authorities, which meant that almost anything could happen, and frequently did. A benign example of this was the setting up of the excellent progressive mental health charity Core Arts. In 1993, local artist Paul Monks commandeered one of the numerous empty wards and was using it as his own studio. A few patients, wandering around the site looking for saleable items to scavenge, stumbled across him accidentally, and he allowed them to use his materials to create their own work. Things snowballed, and within a few weeks dozens of mad artists were discovering their creativity. Funding was secured, a recording studio was added, and Core Arts went on to find its own premises and go from strength to strength. Quite separately, an art exhibition – *Rear Window* – took shape across the hospital grounds as they were cleared, and work by famous names like Derek Jarman co-existed with pieces by many survivor artists. These initiatives deservedly met with widespread acclaim, though our own received a more guarded welcome.

Phil Murphy drafted a constitution for the Patients Council and money was raised from the local Health Authority, which was responding to the burgeoning London-wide call for 'user groups' to be taken seriously. Ironically this demand was helped by Thatcher's drive for people in hospitals to be treated as 'consumers' rather than 'patients', as part of a strategy to bring healthcare into the realm of the free market. Hopefully Thatcher will be turning in her grave as she realises some of the results of this 'consumerism'. Roger, City and Hackney Mind's redoubtable director, helped with our funding negotiations. Debates have taken place within the user movement over the potential conflict of interests if user groups or advocacy services are funded by statutory bodies like Health Authorities, which will be running many of the services user groups complain about. The fear is that groups will be threatened with withdrawal of funding unless they shut up about sensitive issues. Although in theory this is a possibility, it's never actually happened with anything I've ever been involved with, and if anyone is willing to throw money at projects I work for, I'm cautious but happy.

The structure of Hackney Patients Council was to some extent misconceived. It was envisaged that there would be four workers, each working ten hours a week for a tenner an hour, with at least one black and female worker. Looking back, we'd have been better off recruiting one very skilled full-time worker to hold the show together from a central position. As it was, the fact that the arrangement was incompatible with most users' welfare benefits situations, and the time the workers spent communicating with each other in team meetings quadrupling the time it took to do anything, helped lay the foundations for the Council turning much later into an irrelevance, which the local mental health trust managers could use to make it appear that users were being consulted, without having to deal with the challenges that would arise if this was really the case.

Things were fine at first: full of optimism, energy, humour and genuinely constructive work. Phil Murphy was one of the four recruited. The others were Andy Martin from anarcho-punk terrors the Apostles; Julie Hathaway, who I'd met when she was a patient at the day ward the Junction; and Alan Dennis, who immediately failed to endear himself to the other Patients Council and advocacy workers by reading the *Daily Sport* in front of everyone, staring at the pictures of naked women brazenly in the office whenever there was a break in the work.

A system was instigated by Phil whereby each worker would visit designated wards weekly, talk with the current inpatients, and record the comments they made both positive and negative, using them to compile data which could then be used to lobby the Health Authority and nursing management for improvements in the patients' material and social conditions.

One of the problems was that, though it was easy enough to convince senior management bureaucrats to agree to changes concerning specific issues, it was hard to get these agreements to filter down to practice on the hospital floor. Power didn't work that way, and by the time policy decisions passed through several different hierarchical strata of professionals, they frequently became meaningless. For example, after the wards had moved from the old Hackney hospital to the new Homerton building and PICU was re-branded Bevan Ward – presumably to stay one step ahead of the horror and stigma associated with the name 'PICU' in the same way that Windscale changed its name to Sellafield – visitors to the ward were banned unless they were social workers or lawyers. A sign had appeared outside reading *"no visitors except close relatives"*, and even close relatives began, suddenly, to find their visits restricted, curtailed or even non-existent, whilst mere friends could just forget it. Senior management agreed to remove the sign and restore patients' visiting rights; however, it took more than a year for the sign to be removed, and still longer before nurses stopped enforcing the restrictions.

Another problem with PICU, or Bevan Ward, where patients were guaranteed the harshest treatment, was race. A continual cat-and-mouse game was fought concerning the slammer, as I called it, and the fact that it was almost exclusively the domain of young male African Caribbean patients, who the doctors and nurses seemed scared of apparently because of their skin colour. This was bad enough, and too frequently one lone woman would be sent to the slammer, which would be intimidating for them as they would literally be the only female on the ward. The Patients Council lobbied for years for Bevan to be a designated men-only ward, and hospital management from time to time ceded to this demand only to change their minds a little while later, whenever a lone woman appeared on one of the other wards who staff found a bit of a handful. I'm not making light of the plight of the black guys, who were often there only because of racist stereotyping and who were often subject to gratuitous and unnecessary forensic assessments to determine the 'likelihood' of them becoming criminals, leading some to private hospitals and special hospitals like Broadmoor with little chance of getting out. Private hospitals in particular had a financial motive for keeping hold of their patients, so that they could continue to charge exorbitant sums of money to the Health Authorities who had sent them. These places had a vested interest in patients not recovering. Robert Jones was in one such hospital, Kneesworth House in Hertfordshire.

Kneesworth had a policy of 'intensive environment therapy', a phrase meaning overcrowded wards. The more patients they had, the more money they could charge, and the phrase was a way of pretending that this was in fact for the patients' own good. Robert was a troublemaker of the best kind, who I'd first met in the small forensic ward at the old Hackney hospital and who was transferred to Kneesworth as part of his ongoing 'rehabilitation'. He'd torched a few schools in the past, but by the time I met him, he was well and had seen the error of his ways. He knew how to work the media, and kept tipping off *Guardian* and *Observer* journalists about scandals he came across in hospitals he was in. Most often papers picked up on deaths of hospital patients which had been covered up. Deaths apparently caused by overdoses of forced anti-psychotic drugs were common in Kneesworth, and staff would pull ranks to disguise or mitigate the circumstances of what may have been medical murders. Initially the hospital retaliated by stopping all of Robert's medication in one go, hoping that the withdrawal symptoms would prove so severe that he'd lose the plot really badly, withdrawal symptoms routinely being dismissed within the psychiatric profession as part of the illness

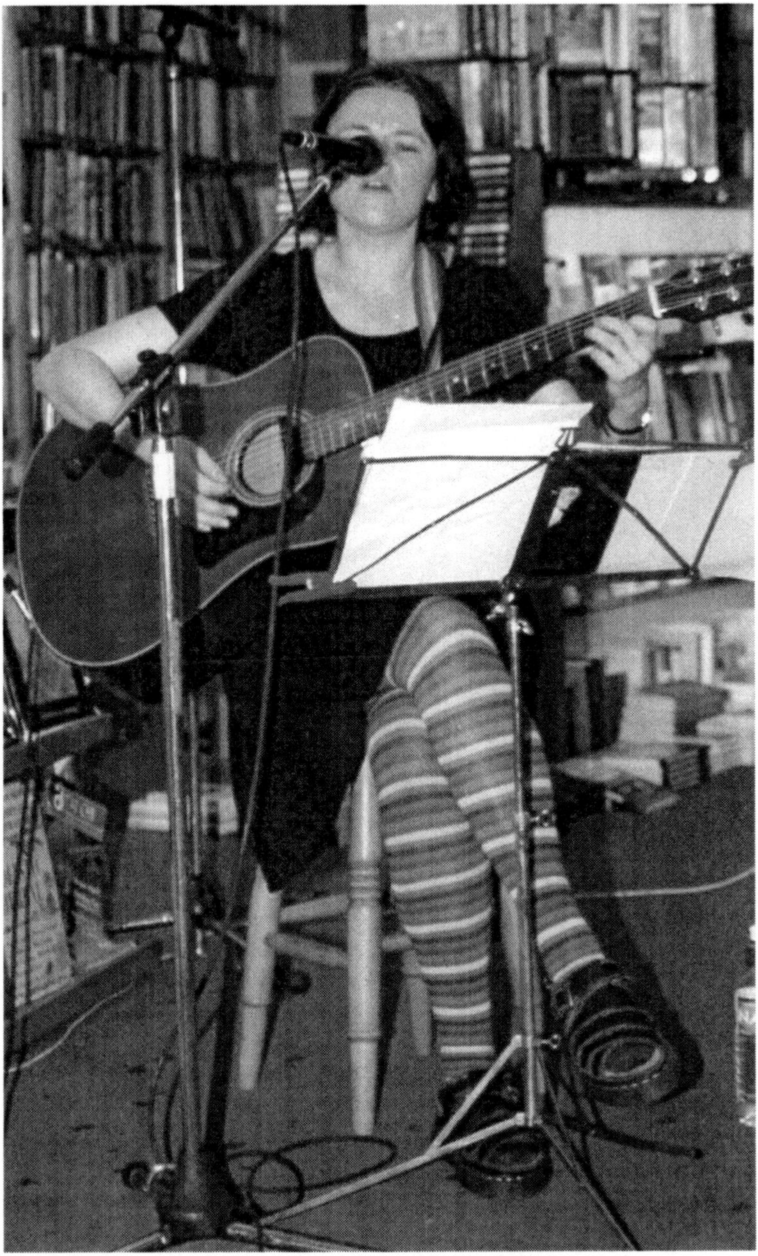

Julie Hathaway, at the launch of the Mad Pride anthology, Compendium Books, Camden, May 2000

the drugs were suppressing in the first place. The strategy was to get him shunted off to Broadmoor for the rest of his life by way of revenge, to set an example to other patients. But Robert got away with his bravery, and managed to stay sane. After several years, he was released.

One man who it seemed would never be released was historian EP Thompson's grandson Tim, who wrote a lengthy chapter for the *Mad Pride* anthology. Incarcerated from the age of sixteen, he spent many years being moved from hospital to hospital, including a long spell at Kneesworth. Whenever I saw him seen him he seemed all right, and he could probably have had a life in the community and been able to cope quite well given the right support. Medical staff claimed that he was too institutionalised to cope with the outside world, which seemed to me to represent something of a conundrum.

The first major success for the Patients Council was a launch party in the advocacy office in the evacuated ECT suite on the ground floor of F block. The new office was near to the Junction, a day ward offering therapeutic and psychological interventions on top of straightforward psychiatry, and whose staff we got on with reasonably well. For the party, which took place on November the fifth, we spent a fortune on food and fireworks, and made several trips to the off licence to stock up on booze. We were lucky to be in contact with top sculptor Keith 'Mally' Mallinson, who took advantage of F block's lax security to climb the stairs to Connolly Ward on the top floor, where he discreetly observed Dr Trevor Turner, the controversial consultant psychiatrist for the south east quarter of Hackney, showing the junior shrinks how it was done in his ward round. Mally got out his notepad and sketched a reasonable likeness of the doctor.

On the day of the party, Mally and Earil gathered a collection of wooden pallets and other debris from the site of the Medium Secure Unit being built nearby. A tall pile of inflammable material grew outside the nurses' home, a building on the hospital grounds still occupied by poorly paid junior nurses living in box rooms. Meanwhile the advocacy office and adjacent disused rooms began to teem with current and former patients.

Nearly all of the inpatients who were allowed out unescorted had turned up, and they were knocking back the abundant supply of beer and wine. Animated chatter competed for audibility with the ghetto blaster pounding out non-stop reggae and soul.

Surprisingly this went on for some hours unchallenged by hospital staff, despite a few curious nurses wandering in and helping themselves to the booze, asking us not to grass them up to the ward managers. You would have assumed that it was a normal house party if it wasn't for the fact that many of the patients wore hospital pyjamas.

The party wore on, the booze kicked in, and two impressive artworks were revealed. The first was a tall, colourful portrait of Dr Turner, painted with oils in Paul Monks' studio by Jim Cleghorn. The masterpiece, entitled *The Doctor of My Dreams*, depicted the shrink naked except for stockings and suspenders. Next, Mally's creation was revealed: sat on a chair, the patients council 'guy', a life-size and remarkably accurate effigy of Dr Turner made out of papier mache and other materials, complete with suit, tie, spectacles and clinical gaze checking for symptoms.

Unfortunately, the hospital site co-ordinator found out about the wooden heap that had appeared outside the nurses' home and she made several frantic and concerned telephone calls to the advocacy office while the party was in full swing. For some reason, she had this idea that we were planning a bonfire later. After being threatened with the police unless we backed down, a compromise was reached and we were permitted to set off our fireworks, but with no bonfire.

Outside, darkness drew in early, and reports reached the party of drunken, disordered behaviour at the wards on the above floors. One or two patients had puked and the nurses had had to clear it up. Also many were in a good mood, being unusually boisterous and giving the nurses a hard time. Several bottles of wine were confiscated.

Leaving Trevor in his chair, we announced that the party was moving to the tarmac outside the nurses' home. The pyre was still there but would remain unlit, giving the effigy a reprieve. In the small garden area next to the staff residential quarters, fresh fireworks were planted: no expense had been spared and most of them were more than a foot long. Showers of stars and sparks in glorious rainbow colours cascaded into the sky above as a succession of roman candles, catherine wheels and fizzy volcanoes held the audience's attention. One or two nurses came out to watch but behaved themselves and didn't interfere.

Each firework seemed somehow bigger than the one before, and in the growing excitement we set off more and more of them in one go each time. Snaps, crackles and pops thundered loudly, defiant and somehow eerie, across the hospital grounds, fierce explosions echoing and ricocheting against the nineteenth century buildings. Finally we were down to the last firework, a rocket, which was nearly seven feet long including its stalk!

We didn't have a milk bottle big enough to launch it from, but eventually we found a suitable litter bin. Mally lit the touchpaper and we all stood back. Hushed expectancy mingled with trepidation: it was the biggest firework any of us had ever seen!

After what seemed like ages the rocket took off and flew gloriously into space, sparkling and shining like the brightest shooting star before hitting its climax: a nuclear explosion, multi-coloured sheets of lightning turning the sky from dark to light for miles around. Chaos escalated and there were scenes unseen in East London since the blitz. Throughout the square half-mile of the hospital grounds, from each wall of every building, bright, blinding bulbs flashed wildly: brilliant, high-powered lights we hadn't known were there. It wasn't dark anymore: in fact, the deranged glare was completely overwhelming. At the same time, an air raid siren pierced the atmosphere at a volume of hundreds of decibels, its source seemingly from every molecule of matter in the grounds; deafening and ghastly. Those of us loosely responsible for organising the party decided it was time to make ourselves scarce and go to the pub. Rushing back to where the party had been to collect our belongings, we encountered a gang of domestics and nurses stampeding down the stairs in panic. Mistakenly, they thought that the fire alarms had been set off by patients smoking dope in the toilets. They weren't too pleased. Trying to look innocent we got our stuff and left, in time to witness a dozen fire engines all speeding into the hospital grounds. It wasn't me, Sir.

The effigy of Dr Turner sat in the advocacy office for a fortnight until an arrangement was made to burn him in a neighbour's back garden. Turner was thrown onto the grass, petrol was sprayed over him and then the bastard was set alight. Watching the establishment pillar and controversial authority figure go up in flames was a truly moving and heart-warming experience for the several dozen spectators. A number of bangers and fireworks had been inserted into the psychiatrist's body, and they exploded in fits and starts as the cremation took its course. The doctor's bones weren't made out of any old rubbish, they were good quality stuff: firm, solid wood that combusted at its own pace without losing any spectacular effect. The wood had been carved into the exact shape of a human skeleton, and as the flesh began to melt and drip away, a perfect bone structure was revealed and glowed a pleasant shade of red as the doctor decomposed: the rib-cage was especially splendid. The event became an occult ceremony: several spectators pissed ritually over the embers and some hocus-pocus was uttered. We imagined that the real doctor would fail to appear at work the following day. Finally the fire burnt out and all that was left of the eminent professional was the lower part of one of his legs, still wearing a smart and polished shoe.

After this, Dave Fanning from the Apostles produced a firecracker incorporating no fewer than 750 bangers, including some huge ones nearly as large as the missile that had struck the hospital barely two weeks earlier. There were children's swings at the end of the garden and Dave attached the firecracker cautiously to the frame. Making sure that the crowd stood well back, Dave held his lighter at arm's length, lit the touchpaper and ran like fuck. There was a lengthy succession of ever-loudening explosions as the flame manoeuvred its way around the maze of fuse: thundering and cacophonous, the sound of the sky itself crashing to the ground: the apocalypse!

As soon as the sonic attack ceased, frenzied shouting erupted across the neighbourhood and the people in the flats opposite peered, afraid, from behind their net curtains. And then the sirens: police cars, ambulances, fire engines – the lot. Surprisingly they pulled up outside a house down the road and it was several minutes before they picked on us. We pretended to be sensible. It transpired that the vibrations caused by the giant firecracker had caused the roof of a nearby house to collapse.

Somehow we fronted it out: indeed, it seemed at the time that we could get away with anything. Sometimes this took the form of photocopied material circulated anonymously around the hospital and beyond. I designed a board game, *Escape From PICU,* which involved dice, and players sent back or forward several squares for encountering God, Satan, heavy handed nurses, and doctors in Nazi uniforms sodomising one another, in true snakes and ladders fashion. The winner encountered freedom in the hospitable form of the Samuel Pepys, a popular local pub. Another venture was a single issue of the magazine *Kommunity*

Kare which I compiled with Dan McQuillan, and which made the official Patients Council magazine *Time In* look like the *Daily Mail*. Encompassing issues around learning difficulties as well as mental health, it contained headlines like "*fuck hospitals*" and "*SANE: fucking cunts*" with a picture of a gun being held to SANE chief executive Marjorie Wallace's head.

Two other events, which would be unfeasible now in any psychiatric institution, occurred shortly after. The first was a punk rock concert on Rainbow Ward, an acute unit on the second floor of F block. Somehow we managed to persuade nursing management that it was okay for us to put on the Apostles, by then called Academy 23, and a one-off Phil Murphy incarnation called Section 3 on the same bill in front of dozens of inpatients.

Prior to all of this, early on in my work in Hackney I'd met Frank Bangay, and a mutual love of similar musicians helped lead to a friendship. He'd co-founded Survivors' Poetry with Peter Campbell, Joe Bidder and others in the early 1990s, an organisation initially devoted to promoting grass-roots poetry and music events by survivors of mental distress, using day centres, community residential units and estate halls as venues. I went to many of their early monthly shows in a community centre in Euston, and found them very inspiring. Although the atmosphere there was quiet and safe, reflecting in part institutional conventions, it was clear that many people were empowered by their involvement and some great poetry came out of it, as evidenced by the anthologies *From Dark to Light* and *Under the Asylum Tree*. As the organisation grew and funding was procured, the ethos necessarily became more professional and less alternative. But for a while Survivors Poetry was calmly phenomenal as an expression of underground creativity, and it was an important chapter in the history of the user movement.

I'd known dozens of mad punk musicians since I was fifteen. It occurred to me that if we could have survivors' poetry, then why not survivors' punk rock? People I mentioned this idea to at the time thought it ridiculous, and certainly the likes of the Apostles and Rudimentary Peni might have scared the living daylights out of a typical monthly Survivors' Poetry audience and had half of them running off to the nearest psychiatric accident and emergency clinic. It wasn't until 1999 that the doubters were seriously proved wrong, but the Rainbow concert was an important milestone. The patients in the audience loved it, even though the staff were intimidated and confused. And we didn't even need to worry about the music distressing people, because nurses were on hand whose job it was to deal with it.

Phil's four-piece rock band kicked off the evening with a selection of cover versions of songs by the New York Dolls, Neil Young, Blur and Roxy Music, as well as two of Phil's new compositions which were very much in the same heartbreakingly harmonious vein as his 1980s band the Regular Guys, moving some to tears. Those of us who'd seen Phil sing and play guitar before knew pretty much what to expect and simply felt sad that his shyness prevented him from performing more often. The rest of the crowd didn't know what had hit them; it was a strange place for such powerful, professional and intense rock to be aired.

The Apostles came next with a maverick, tuneful set which endeared Andy to the on-looking lunatics enormously. Andy at the time deluded himself that his band sounded like Emerson Lake and Palmer, but in fact it was simply generic, lumpen anarcho-punk at its best. The final song in the set was the mid-1980s indie chart-topper 'Mob Violence', which goes: "*The only thing I know that makes me feel high/ is a half brick landing in a copper's eye/ the only thing I know that makes me feel nice/ is the sight and sound of an incendiary device/ mob violence! Mob violence!/ fists and faces meet when we take to the street/ mob violence! Mob violence!/ because we get our kicks throwing bottles and bricks/ mob violence! Mob violence!/ class anger exploded when we take to the roads*" and so on. The patients knew what Andy meant, but the hospital security guards who wandered into the ward to see what was going on midway during the song seemed bemused, and the nurses were distinctly uncomfortable.

Miraculously another party followed, to coincide with the final demise of the Hackney Hospital and the relocation of its wards to the new gaff round the corner. This party was ostensibly a joint effort organised by the Rainbow nursing staff with Hackney Patients Council to usher in a new spirit of co-operation as, 266 years after Hackney Poor House first opened, the institution reached its final night. Big Steve from Core Arts and later the Arlenes did a set of Elvis covers with his mates, and various Survivors' Poetry Poetry stalwarts performed. But sadly the attempted partnership failed as the senior Rainbow nurse became distressed by Council members' drinking and swearing. Using her walkie-talkie, she 'bleeped' her immediate superior for the night, the pregnant-woman-restraining Dennis Drake. He was pleased to spoil the fun by bringing the party to a premature end.

Questions were asked later. Whenever a Patients Council event took place, staff, especially middle management, always wanted to know who was in charge. They'd been so thoroughly indoctrinated with the hierarchical structure of nursing that they thought it inconceivable that anything could ever function otherwise. *"Nobody's in charge, we all take responsibility"* we once told a baffled ward manager Shaun Hare. *"I'm sorry, I don't get you"* he replied, scratching his head. He genuinely hadn't a clue what we were going on about.

It was good that the hospital was closing down, but it was kind of sad to explore the corridors, wards and offices of the deserted blocks. A disinterested observer might have concluded that the place had been colonised by junkies, but in fact the syringes scattered liberally across the floors had all been left behind by the medical staff. There were rubber gloves, medical records, ECT machines, desks, tables, filing cabinets, iron lungs, scalpels, stethoscopes, straightjackets and all sorts of other paraphernalia: a treasure-trove of clinical waste. Heartbreakingly one of the empty wards, a forgotten psychogeriatric unit, was filled to the ceiling with forgotten paintings representing perhaps the final testaments of their creators, discarded and dumped just as the painters and their predecessors had been discarded and dumped into the Hackney Hospital. Faces, landscapes and abstract images, some unbelievably bleak, all destined to be crushed beneath the bulldozers along with the hollow tombstone in which they lay abandoned.

It had been talked about and delayed for so long that nobody thought it would really happen. But one day F block had four wards full of patients and by the next, following the previous night's prematurely curtailed party, everyone was gone save for a few security guards and hangers-on from the arts projects mentioned earlier. A lot of equipment was left behind, and I managed to scavenge a fridge from one of the empty wards. I'd destroyed my previous one on the same day, trying to defrost it by scraping at the freezer compartment with a knife. I'd never thought about how fridges worked, and it was a surprise when toxic gas started to hiss from the wound my blade had cut into the lining. Paul Monks ended up with a fridge too, and many other workers at the hospital stocked up on various household items.

The new hospital around the corner was exactly the same as the old one, only newer and more efficient. There were now very few holes in the institutional armour, and spy cameras were everywhere. For a few days after it opened, the security staff couldn't stop looking at the monitors in their office. They couldn't believe it: all that vision and power. They were charging around the unit reacting to the slightest hint of misdemeanour, challenging people urinating in the corridors or smoking in the wrong place. And then the novelty wore off and things settled down.

But back in 1994, the most urgent preoccupation of Hackney Patients Council was football.

Terry Conway, who had become the council's chair, had dozens of friends who played in the upper echelons of non-league football. He decided to knock Hackney Patients Council into proper shape as a team, challenging the nursing staff to an eleven-a-side game over ninety minutes on Hackney Marshes. Obviously this was a game we had to win at all costs, to avoid losing face. A few genuine hospital faces were in our team including Phil, Earil and myself in defence, Terry in midfield and Elaine Shapiro operating up front. But Terry had also recruited several top ringers, and the wankers on the other side were completely humiliated. The ringers were straight-faced and conscientious as they described the depressing details of their fictitious hospital admissions, and we stuffed the nurses 12-2. The staff couldn't believe it; it was the worst thing that had ever happened to them. They were walking around with their heads hung miserably, hoping that nobody would recognise them for weeks afterwards.

Elaine was a laugh. Once, when manic, she trashed Shaun Hare's car and scrawled *"You've got AIDS"* across the windscreen with lipstick. She came into our office and told us about it.

"That's not funny!" Julie Hathaway protested, earnestly. *"No, it's not"*, I agreed. Then simultaneously we realised that it was funny after all and fell about laughing helplessly. We were a bunch of bastards in those days.

The next match was against Broadmoor. For obvious reasons, it had to be an away fixture. We were part of a tournament with several teams involved, and as we had less of a point to prove against Broadmoor we fielded a weaker squad, which included myself, Terry, Phil, Jo Crane, Debbie McNamara and others. We were knocked out of the tournament after a few games.

We didn't care. Against the nurses it had been the winning that counted, not the taking part, but this time the reverse was true.

To get to Broadmoor's sports stadium we had to pass through several locked doors and partitions, and we were scanned by X-ray machines and monitored for radiation. High solid steel fences topped with barbed wire surrounded the field, and in each corner there was a turret occupied by guards wearing vintage Nazi uniforms showing off rifles ready to shoot anyone who tried to escape. Between games I got chatting to an interesting and pleasant spectator named Robert Hunter, who was in for blowing up Greater Manchester police station with dynamite. The explosion had killed seven old bill, and he wasn't due to be considered for release until 2010 at the very earliest. The cull of police wasn't widely known because it was subject to a government D-notice, disallowing media reportage.

"There were ten coppers in there", Robert explained, *"and three got out alive. Luckily though, I got the one I wanted, the chief superintendent, who was my dad. He'd been knocking my old dear about for a while and of course, something had to be done. I'd have been really upset if he'd been one of the cops who'd walked. I was criticised afterwards, because some people don't like dynamite. They say it's old-fashioned, and gelignite is better. But I'm not sure I agree: I think dynamite's all right. It might not really be rated these days, but it gets the job done."*

It's illegal for security reasons to take photographs in Broadmoor, but nevertheless I still have a team picture of us that was taken there. I put it on my living room wall after Jo died in 1999, then after a while this seemed too sad so I took it down.

The hospital moved in 1994, and we were at first relocated to a room in the psychiatric emergency clinic. One wall consisted entirely of a two-way mirror compromising our privacy, so I concealed it with an old sheet. Then after some lobbying we were moved to a room directly opposite the new Connolly ward with two other wards in the same corridor. Here, as I intended, we were immediately accessible to all of the inpatients who were banging on the door non-stop with usually pertinent requests, and it was pressure. Sasere couldn't handle it and began spending the majority of her time in City and Hackney Mind's main offices to escape from the crossfire. Me, Hatice the Turkish advocate and a small gang of volunteers were left to deal with the flood of horror with our backs to the wall. Unbelievably, Leila Salim chose to work in this difficult atmosphere almost full-time

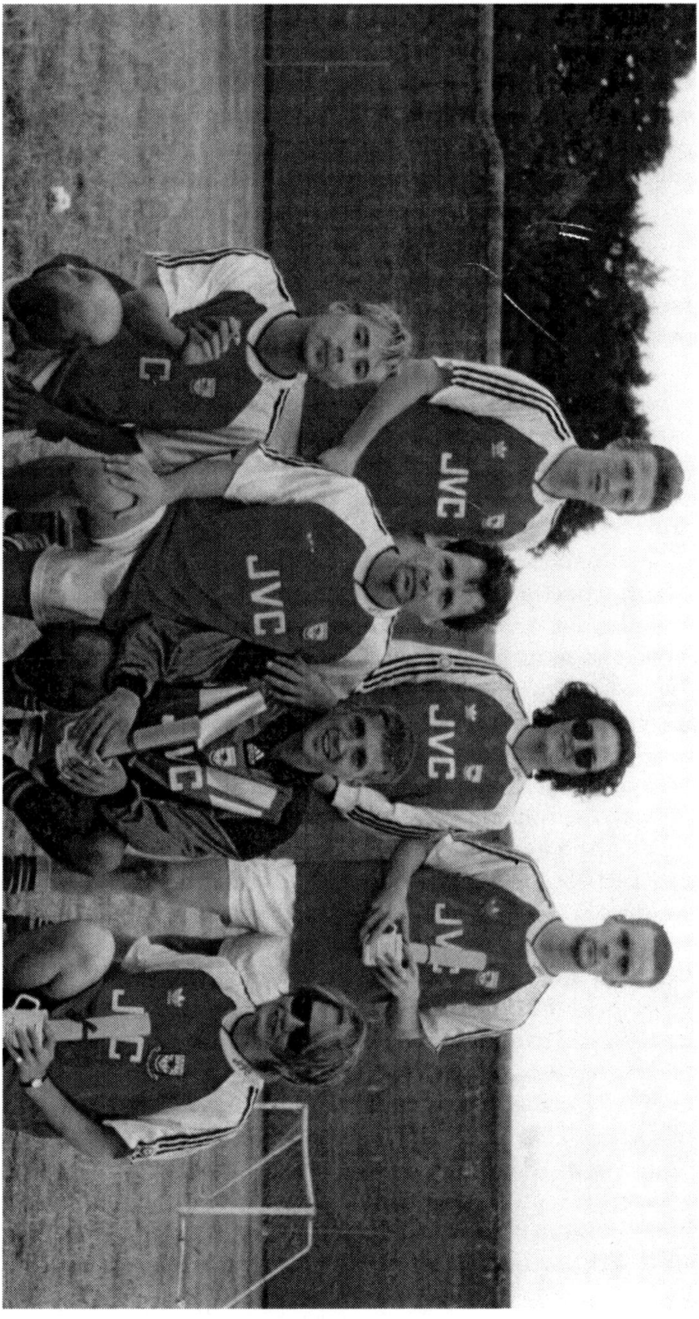

Hackney Patients Council 5-a-side squad at Broadmoor in 1994. Photo Taken illegally, cameras not being allowed. Back Row: unkown, Debbie McNamara, unkown. Front Row: Rob Dellar, Terry Conway, unkown, Jo Crane

without being paid, performing administration tasks and individual advocacy, and helping to cover for the idiosyncrasies of the paid staff. I've no idea how we'd have managed without her and I wonder how many other unsung heroes keep high-profile projects on the go from behind the scenes. Between us the work got done and the service was popular with the patients, although one satisfied customer saw fit to scrawl *"FUCKING BASTARDS, CUNTS"* across our office door in black marker pen. I left the graffiti there and surrounded it with pictures of Princess Margaret, who had recently died, one of the hospital doctors and other people I disliked.

The Patients Council got an office at the other end of the corridor a little later, but the effectiveness of the group was already beginning to wane. Julie, the most stable of the workers, left to become an occupational therapist. At one point we were supposed to raise match-funding to create a full-time co-ordinator post, after the King's Fund agreed to pay for half of it if another organisation coughed up for the other half. Phil, his mental health worsening, became obsessed with the idea that the post-holder should not be someone who had used mental health services, and most of the rest of us disagreed. Instead of concentrating on fundraising we became sidetracked by arguing about this issue, and consequently the post never came to exist. I managed to put an application to the Barings Foundation, but this group collapsed before the form was processed, courtesy of rogue trader Nick Leeson. He grew up in the same area of Watford as I did, though he was a year younger than me and I never met the scumbag. Debbie McNamara replaced Julie and sporadically did some good work. Andy's conduct became increasingly bizarre. He'd sit in the patients council office all day using the computer to write polemics and articles about physics and astronomy regurgitated from archaic text books he'd read and pretended to understand. Some interesting magazines came out of this, but nothing useful for the psychiatric patients he was paid to work with. On one occasion, he presented us with an article ostensibly written for our magazine *Time In* by Alan, a young patient he liked. Written in Andy's distinctive, literary and grammatically flawless style, the article presented some interesting observations about hospital life, although Alan couldn't remember a thing about the piece when asked about it while attending a literacy class at Tudor Road, learning how to read and write.

There were still some laughs to be had. In 1995 the Patients Council held an away weekend in Avebury, Wiltshire. The village was a magnet for hippies because it had a top ancient stone circle in it which made Stonehenge look like a couple of bollards at the edge of a council estate in Hackney. Also it had West Kennett Long Barrow which was some kind of prehistoric crypt, and Silbury Hill, the tallest man-made hill in Britain which was put there a few millennia ago for no apparent reason, and which looked distinctly mammary, especially if someone pitched a tent directly on top of it. I had a friend who lived there, Emma McElwee. Except for Phil and Andy who disliked travelling, we all descended on the druidic paradise on the same day as King Arthur. Arthur Pendragon, who believed himself to be the reincarnation of the original king, was a former Hell's Angel who was often arrested for carrying an offensive weapon in public: his ceremonial sword, Excalibur. Sean O'Reilly, who became chair of Southwark Mind, was once in the same prison as this daft twat. At one point the cops confiscated the sword and threatened to melt it down, but after an appeal Arthur was allowed to keep it on 'religious' grounds.

We were trying to have a picnic and kick a ball around. King Arthur and his mates turned up and held a pagan ritual in a nearby field, dispersing some of the local sheep. Two hundred hippies stood in a circle chanting *"King Arthur is coming!"* in response to whatever rubbish emanated from Pendragon's mouth. The sheep sometimes disrupted the circle by strolling in and out of it and bleating.

"Fucking weirdoes!" Jo Crane observed, kicking a football towards the circle and missing the King's head by inches. It was nice for us to be able to patronise people crazier than us for a change.

Some of the characters the Patients Council attracted onto its management committee were colourful, though not all of them lasted too long as some were intimidated by the actions of the staff and afraid to challenge them. Dan McQuillan was treasurer at one point but resigned after being shouted at by Phil; others fell by the wayside, put off by what was perceived as a bunker mentality amongst the workers, who resented being given any advice or instructions increasingly as time went by. Deb Percy, another treasurer, was colourful. She'd been a bureaucrat with City and East London Health Authority but was interested in patients' rights and attracted by the spirit of rebellion we exuded. Bored with her job, she resigned and became a professional dominatrix, which made waves. At a meeting with nursing staff, Deb was referred to by manager Jim Keown as *"that awful woman"*. He was something of a square, and judgemental about her career choice. Our response was *"hey, that's our mate you're talking about"*.

A character who really was dodgy was Paul Turner, who succeeded Terry as management committee chair after Terry's social work career took off. Paul was a Green party councillor in Stoke Newington introduced to the Patients Council by fellow Green activist Julie. His local political profile meant that, when he was charged with downloading kiddie porn from the internet and sharing it with other paedophiles, it immediately made the front page of the *Hackney Gazette* with a big picture of him looking sleazy. Bizarrely and without discussing it with anyone, Andy issued a statement on behalf of the Patients Council affirming that Paul was innocent of all charges, even though he had previous and had already pleaded guilty. After the nonce came out of prison, he expected to resume his position as chair. Debbie phoned me asking my opinion regarding whether this would be a wise move, Paul having in fact done a sterling job for us. *"No way"*, I advised her. *"Can you imagine the headline of the next* Hackney Gazette*? Hello, hello I'm back again!"*

My advice was heeded, which was just as well because it wasn't long before Paul was back behind bars for doing the same thing again. Other Patients Council allies included community development expert Arun Mushiana, and a succession of real or fictitious Chinese and Vietnamese characters recruited or invented by Andy. But the game was up, people left, and by the 21st century Hackney Patients Council was nothing more than a front for Andy to be paid by the Health Authority to pursue his own projects unrelated to mental health issues, and in turn for the Health Authority to pretend to be funding user involvement, an arrangement which suited both parties. We'd made plenty of mistakes, but I would put the lessons I'd learnt to good use later.

Fairy Tale in the Supermarket

It was autumn 1994 when I decided to give up smoking cannabis, having spent the entirety of my late teens and twenties under the influence of the stuff from the moment I woke up until I passed out at night. Some people argue that cannabis isn't addictive, but the withdrawal symptoms were real enough, if not unpleasant, and I entered into a controlled mania lasting several months. A berserk energy was unleashed, which I compensated for in part by increasing my alcohol consumption without realising at the time. I felt higher than I ever had when stoned, and an avalanche of creative ideas tumbled into my head; I even painted some pictures, which were dreadful.

My friend Nick Blinko of Rudimentary Peni had written a semi-autobiographical novel, *The Primal Screamer,* about primal scream therapy and punk rock. Reading the manuscript he'd sent me, I recognised it instantly as a classic and sent copies to various publishers hoping to get Nick a deal. The copies were sent back with standard covering rejection letters, although Ramsay Kanaan from anarchist publisher and distributor AK Press later admitted he had 'egg on his face' for doubting the novel. I decided to publish the fucker myself, surmising that there was a gap in the market for good quality 'mad' literature that no other publishers would touch. *The Primal Screamer* became the first release of the Spare Change Books imprint and it was an instant hit. Nick had also written a book of short stories, but unfortunately he couldn't remember where he'd put them.

Nick is an interesting guy who has had some fantastic delusions. His paintings, which have been exhibited all over the world and earned him legendary status in the outsider art scene, consist of microscopically detailed images of tortured faces, figures, twisted fantasy creatures, and as he describes it, *"visual representations of suicidal depression"*. He buried one of these artworks in his dad's back garden, believing that a plant would grow there that would visually resemble the painting. Sadly, he was wrong.

In 1987, Nick recorded Rudimentary Peni's best album *Cacophony,* which used imagery drawn from the works of HP Lovecraft to cleverly chronicle the psychotic breakdown he was having at the time. When the album was finished he was carted off to the psychiatric ward at Watford General Hospital, whose other notable occupants have included Geri Halliwell, and Poly Styrene from X-Ray Spex. Nick believed that, as a sacrifice to his remarkable and disturbing album, he'd recruited several rock stars to add backing vocals or guitar solos to the record and then he'd killed them all.

This is how Nick killed Elton John. After Sir Elton performed a piano solo which ended up adorning one of *Cacophony*'s tracks, Elton was shagging Nick up the arse on the floor of the recording studio, until Nick managed to use his arse muscles to yank off Elton's cock leaving the pianist to bleed to death, dickless and in agony on the studio floor. Poor old Elton: his hits haven't sounded the same since, probably because the lookalike recruited by his record company to fill the void hasn't quite the same genius and charisma as the original bespectacled slaphead.

Cacophony was eventually released in 1989 to widespread acclaim. Nick's next record was *Pope Adrian 37th Psychristiatric,* released in 1995 to coincide with *The Primal Screamer.* Nick had convinced himself that he was in fact the pope. From his hospital cubicle he wrote an album's worth of hardcore punk numbers from the holy leader's perspective, and he managed to convince the hospital staff to allow him day release to go into a studio and record them. Tracks included 'Pogo Pope', 'We're Gonna Destroy Life the World Gets Higher and Higher', and 'Pills Popes and Potions', a hymn to psychiatric medication.

Still buzzing, I began compiling *Gobbing, Pogoing and Gratuitous Bad Language: An Anthology of Punk Short Stories,* timed to cash in on the upcoming twentieth anniversary of punk. Around this time I was hanging out a great deal with a group of young, creatively motivated refugees from Brighton, including Keith 'Mally' Mallinson, Lucy Williams and Rob Colson, and I found their enthusiasm and energy inspiring. With Ted Curtis, Martin Cooper and Emma McElwee, we set up a writing group to plan the multi-author novel *Seaton Point*. Separately, I hooked up with Dan McQuillan, Jon Active, Jon Eden, German Chris and other anarchists to plan Hackney Anarchy Week, a nine day long borough-wide festival of subversion.

My domestic life wasn't going too well at the time, with Mina becoming increasingly confused and self-preoccupied to the extent that, at times, it felt as if I was working at one hospital and coming home to another. Creative projects were, in part, a respite from this. The fact that Mina had recently taken a job with Mind in Enfield didn't help. Her boss, Alison Bugg, had been the admin co-ordinator at City and Hackney Mind and I'd got on well with Alison before she got a job as Enfield's director, briefed to set up the charity from scratch with money procured by an executive committee. When Alison advertised a post for a community development worker I encouraged Mina to apply, thinking that Alison would be a tolerant line manager.

I was wrong. Alison proved to be out of her depth in her new role, and apparently became jealous of Mina's superior charisma and work skills. Alison took to undermining Mina's work at every opportunity while trying to take credit herself for Mina's achievements. After a while it appeared that Alison was looking for excuses to get Mina out of the job, specifically by deleting Mina's post and replacing it with an identical one with a different job title. Mina's often bizarre behaviour helped provide Alison with ammunition against her, and a bitter battle ensued lasting for years. Mina resigned before anyone could fire her, hooking up with a Unison trade union official, Claire Andrews, to pursue an industrial tribunal claim for constructive dismissal and racial harassment. For the final year of our relationship, this work dispute was almost all Mina was prepared to talk or think about. It obsessed her every waking moment, and she sank into something bordering on psychosis. Andrews encouraged this obsession, becoming something of a guru figure to Mina who was gullible and vulnerable at the time.

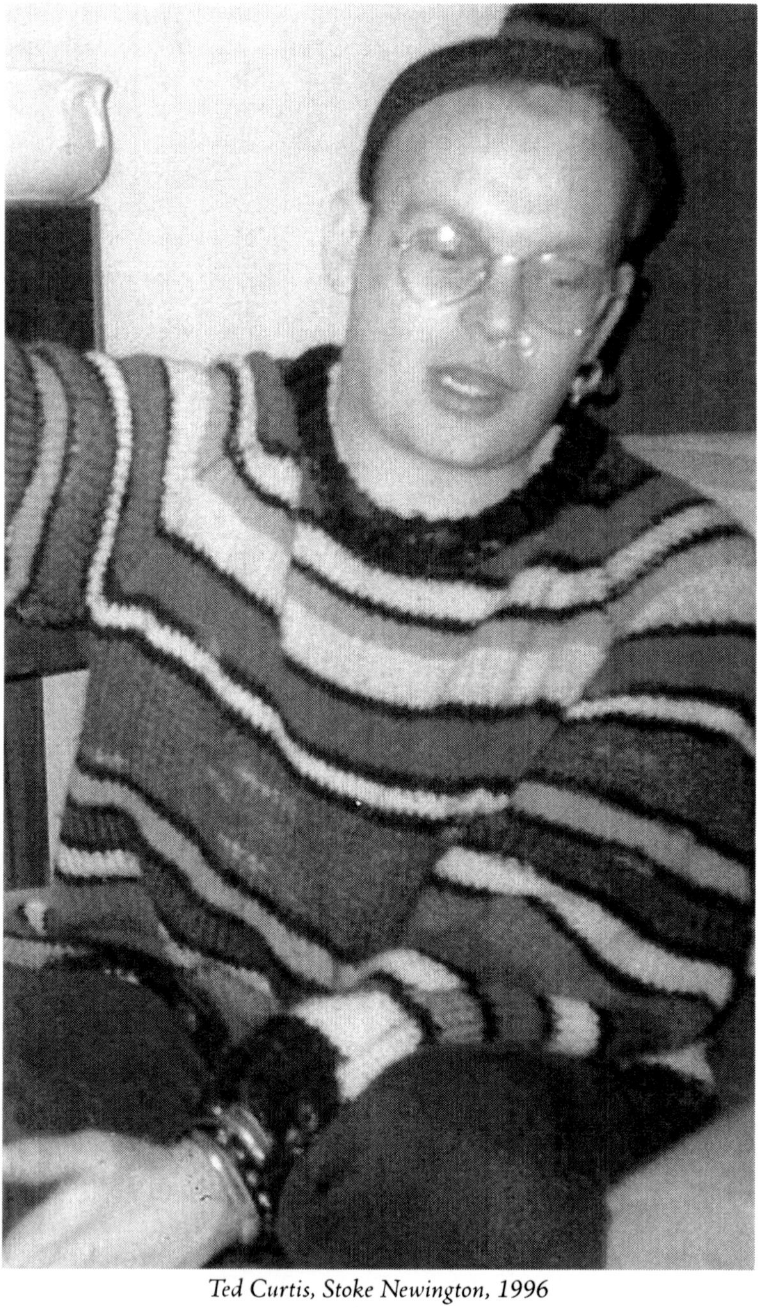

Ted Curtis, Stoke Newington, 1996

Finally Mina walked out on the spur of the moment and took up for a while with Andrews, who was twice her age. Mina eventually won five grand in an out of court settlement, following several tribunal hearings postponed at Andrews' behest for the latter to maintain leverage over her. Andrews made off with the money and the two split up; it transpired that the union official had made a habit of such manipulations.

After twelve years, Mina and myself had split up in April 1996 and I was very badly traumatised. The day before she walked out I had a driving test, my third. I couldn't concentrate: all that I could think about was this suddenly disintegrating relationship, and I failed on a minor technicality. Given what was to come this failure may have been a blessing because driving can be dangerous. On the night she left, I went to Chat's Palace community arts centre in Homerton to watch a show organised by the burgeoning Core Arts, a charity which ironically later gave Mina a job. Blind drunk, I returned home to a note and an empty flat.

By then, some of my previous year's work was reaching fruition. *Gobbing Pogoing and Gratuitous Bad Language* was back from the printers and receiving good reviews. Hackney Anarchy Week was scheduled for a fortnight's time. And my alcohol intake, never moderate at the best of times, escalated further: creative pursuits and heavy drinking seemed at the time the most appropriate ways of numbing my pain. I can remember the day I realised that alcohol had become a chemical addiction. A few days into Hackney Anarchy Week, I came back early one morning to the flat Mina and I had bought together, to feed the cat. I tried to put the needle on my record player down onto a track from one of my favourite albums, *Remember* by Doll By Doll. But my hands were shaking far too much for me to be able to do it.

On the bright side, Hackney had been transformed into an anarchist theme park. Lunatics from all over the world descended onto East London like vultures, and during nine days of fun there were four or five events occurring around the borough at any one time, twenty four hours a day. It was amazing: Hackney didn't know what the fuck had hit it. I have reservations about anarchism these days but once found it attractive and somehow exciting: other anarchist activists were very often charismatic, caring and passionate individuals and a laugh to work with. What little there was of the theory behind anarchism was seductive, appealing to instinctive rebels like me, and its nihilistic aspects somehow mirrored my sense of alienation. It served more as a fashion statement than as a well-considered political or philosophic outlook. In reality the anarchist movement was an incoherent muddle, spanning far-left groups to far-right ones, with people from opposite poles remarkably able to co-operate with each other due to anarchism's barely developed theory. In reality their common ground was often only an 'A' in a circle. Socialist groups tended to be more boring because they spent too much time holding inconsequential meetings and having disputes on the grounds of minor sectarian differences. Socialists were far too sensible and would never have thought of such a happening as Hackney Anarchy Week.

It was a welcome distraction and I was invigilating one of the venues, of all places a church hall: the Barnabas Centre in Homerton Road, where various workshops, a book fair and an art exhibition were held. A worker for the church at one point dismantled Mally's display, considering it blasphemous, which it was, and damaging some of his priceless artworks. Core Arts had recently moved to the back of the building: Paul Monks came out and calmed things down, lecturing the worker about the godlessness of censorship, and the display was restored.

The week kicked off with an opening event at Chat's Palace, the world-famous community arts centre which was unfortunately burnt to the ground somewhere towards the end of *Seaton Point*. Doubling as a launch party for the *Gobbing* anthology, 400 people turned up, twice the capacity dictated by fire regulations. To begin with a guy from the Sisters of Perpetual Indulgence, dressed as a nun, performed an occult ceremony blessing Hackney Anarchy Week and banishing Hackney Council. Then authors from the book gave readings. Emma McElwee scared the anarchists out of their wits with some eerie traditional storytelling. Jess Hopkins declaimed his stuff in so thick a Scottish accent that nobody could understand a word. Stewart Home was heckled as 'sexist' by some of the audience as he deadpanned a sequence from his classic novel *Defiant Pose*, in which a skinhead recites Abeizer Coppe's *A Fiery Flying Roll* while he gets a blow job in a boat floating down the Thames, London simultaneously being destroyed by anarchist rioting. Frank Bangay was very well-received indeed, and he proved that his performance poetry was strong enough to resonate far beyond the coffee houses and Survivors' Poetry ghettos to which he'd been accustomed. And

Phil Murphy, on leave from the psychiatric unit he'd recently wound up in, turned up with a guitar and performed two great songs he'd written. Finally punk legends Alternative TV, augmented by artists who painted murals around them, performed a blistering set of classic punk and avant-garde songs from their early singles and the albums *The Image Has Cracked* and *Vibing Up the Senile Man*. I was very drunk before I even arrived and by the end I was almost comatose, though I can remember Mally approaching me in my stupor and telling me excitedly: "*Nice one! You've done it!*"

A concerned Jon Eden from the Association of Autonomous Astronauts somehow managed to get me in a taxi home, and I arrived back in one piece along with the unsold remainder of the books I'd taken along. The AAA proposed independent, community-led space exploration programmes, as an alternative to the military and business models of space travel promoted by governments. Jon and his mate Richard North from the East London Psychogeographical Association ran a workshop at the Barnabas Centre, leading us all deep into the cosmos.

"*Close your eyes*", Jon told us. Using his occult powers, he cast a spell putting the workshop attendees under his command. "*You are now rising, gently, gradually, towards the ceiling of the church hall. Slowly, you are discovering that the ceiling, and the roof, are merely social constructs to be risen above. And now you escape from these ties, floating gently, gently up, up a little, until you are hovering with the clouds above you, and Homerton High Street below. The people are as ants, and you can see the hospital, the kebab shop, Chat's Palace as insignificant symbols of authority which become smaller as you rise further above Hackney, escaping their rules, even Hackney Empire and the town hall becoming but specks of dust as your liberated spirit throws off its chains, says no to gravity and floats gently, gently into the stratosphere and you can see the whole of London and its twinkling bright lights.*"

After Jon had taken us to the Milky Way and back it was time to play three-sided football. A large map of the moon unfolded onto the floor, and we used it to try to work out routes around Hackney. Tracing the lunar landscape we located a suitable pitch for the match, no further away than the small park squeezed between the Barnabas Centre and Homerton Hospital's psychiatric unit. Three-sided football is a variation on the conventional beautiful game with three teams playing on a hexagonal pitch, with a hole in the middle and three equidistant goalmouths on the outside. Whichever team concedes the least goals wins, which involves allegiances between the teams shifting constantly, making cunning more crucial than ball skills. This has been said to dissolve the homoerotic and homophobic bipolarity of the traditional game, thus undermining the very basis of capitalist organisation. Three-sided football was allegedly invented by former Watford and AC Milan striker Luther Blissett, whose name has been adopted as an alias by several thousands of anarchists over the years, particularly in Italy. Several passing psychiatric patients observed or joined in the match at Homerton, and the result became irrelevant amidst the confusion.

Poetry performances, critical masses, riots, music and sports events: all manner of surrealism engulfed the borough. The Barnabas Centre hosted many workshops. These included Class War debating how best to disrupt the upcoming general election, which would see Tony Blair crowned as the new prime minister; the anarchists reached the conclusion that thousands of stickers needed to be printed bearing slogans along the lines of 'don't vote'. It must have worked, because the constituency of Hackney North and Stoke Newington recorded the lowest turnout in Britain when the election finally came. Only 51 per cent of those on the electoral register could be bothered to vote, and most residents of Hackney weren't even registered.

The McLibel Two, Dave Morris and Helen Steel, ran a group explaining why McDonalds is wrong and describing their legal battle with them. Although I admire the pair immensely, by then I was becoming a little tired of politically correct sanctimony: it was all getting a bit pious. By way of rebellion, I went to McDonalds for the first and only time since childhood and bought a veggieburger the minute the workshop had finished. Two days earlier I'd been part of a group smashing the windows at the outlet. The burger tasted like shit.

Ken Loach delivered a lecture at the Rio cinema in Dalston, and his film *Land and Freedom* was shown. I missed it: I was invigilating the hall where a discussion involving 300 Turkish anarchists was being held. During these events a power cut took place depriving most of Hackney of electricity. The discussion took place in the dark, though fortunately the Rio was just outside the boundary of the grid failure. Sozen Ismail performed most of the interpreting and also turned up at some of the events with food she'd prepared, trying to force me to eat it, as in my trauma and insobriety I'd rarely eaten during the previous fortnight.

Sozen was one of a select few mental health activists on the scene at the time with anarchist sympathies, and the two of us decided to run an 'anarchism and mental health' workshop which we began preparing ten minutes before it was due to start. The preparation involved buying some crayons and a children's colouring book from the nearest shop and rescuing a large cardboard box from a skip. We made the thirty or so workshop participants sit in a circle facing each other, and paced around outside the circle ranting, drawing at best tenuous links between anarchism and mental health. Having satisfied ourselves that the participants were suitably disorientated, we bullied them into colouring in pages from the book using the crayons. On the basis of what they'd created, we forced them each to wear cards bearing the names of the diagnoses we'd given them from our clinical perspective. Spending the next hour with 'schizophrenia', 'borderline personality disorder' and suchlike written on them taught the punters what it was like to be medically labelled.

Then we picked on one unsuspecting punter, put him into the large cardboard box to cut off his vision and make him invisible, and bombarded him with clinical questions to graphically illustrate the power dynamics between practitioners and their patients. The poor guy was terrified and left none the wiser about the relation of anarchism to mental health, except that after the revolution everyone would be mentally more healthy.

I moved out of the flat that I'd shared with Mina, shortly after Mally had split up with Lucy Williams, on his birthday. Mally and his friend Steve Colson needed an extra person in their rented place in Stoke Newington after Lucy moved out. With me as the replacement it was a men behaving badly environment, with heavy round-the-clock drinking, neglect of household chores and general chaos. Upon moving in, on the rebound I hooked up with Sozen Ismail, who by now had 25 cats. She'd become well known for picking up strays from around her estate, the Kingsmead, and trying to find homes for them. Kids would visit her flat and present her with unwanted cats, some of which would breed, and cats accumulated at a faster rate than that at which they could be found homes. I ended up adopting two of them, who Sozen had named 'Magic' and 'Grey One' and whose pictures have appeared on a number of CD sleeves.

Although I felt badly traumatised during this period, there were some good times, including the last occasion I ever took amphetamine sulphate. An opening view was held in South London that night of an exhibition of some of Mally's excellent, humorous sculptures made from found objects, and this was followed later by a launch party in the west end for Nina Antonia's biography of one of my favourite singers, the Only Ones' Peter Perrett, who performed a rare live set. But unfortunately Steve, who had supplied the speed, was busted for it in the early hours of the morning.

Finally the three of us vacated the house early in 1997, by which time rent had become overdue and the place was well trashed, through a combination of our neglect and the landlord's failure to deal with structural defects and repairs. During the three week gap before I could move into my next place, I stayed with Phil Murphy and his then girlfriend Claire at their house in Finsbury Park, from where they were shortly due to be evicted. A large billboard was attached to the side of this house, visible from the passing main road, and the Tories took to sticking posters there asking for people to vote for them in the forthcoming general election. Phil and I got some spray paint and a ladder and amused ourselves by defacing the posters to read: *"Sleazy come, sleazy go"*, a slogan Phil had thought of. Phil, Claire and I went together to the new flat in Lower Clapton when it was time to move, and the couple stayed with me for nine months. I managed to hold down the post of advocacy co-ordinator with City and Hackney Mind through this time, and although I was becoming more chaotic and sometimes intoxicated at work, I was still putting a lot of effort into it and evidently had accumulated some laurels to rest on, and I was getting the job done reasonably well. People around me helped: Leila Salim was vital, often running the office on her own without being paid; and two lawyers, Rod Campbell-Taylor and Jo Richards took on some complex legal work around the Mental Health Act, often working pro bono.

In 1997 Sasere Obaseki left for another job and I never heard from her again, other than for reference requests. Dumisa Morrison took over as African-Caribbean mental health advocate and seemed okay. There came to be a dispute with a member of the Mind staff. Mind had set up a day centre, Homerton Friends Lodge next to the hospital. It catered predominantly for the young black men excluded by most existing day services and it had developed out of an informal drop-in at the old Hackney Hospital site set up by Mind advice officer Lisa Haywood. Len Kerr eventually became manager of the Lodge, which increasingly began to resemble the more institutional day services its target group had found inadequate or inaccessible. Kerr was a flash character in designer clothes, with an expensive wristwatch and gold teeth. He drove a posh car, and he turned up to work when he felt like it talking to his mobile phone, and not doing a lot except for mercilessly disciplining his staff apparently at every opportunity; for example, giving people written warnings for being five minutes late for work. He gained a reputation for hassling women staff and clients, which he no doubt saw as being 'charming', and for generally behaving like the bigshot he believed himself to be. For my part, I'd gained a reputation for filling in DLA forms successfully and, although it wasn't in my job description, I found it difficult to refuse requests for assistance knowing as I did that an income on which it is possible to survive had greater mental health benefits for individuals than all the services put together that the borough of Hackney had to offer. It was getting out of hand, and I tried to show other people how to fill the forms in to share the workload. But after Dumisa did a good job completing a reapplication form for a woman who attended the Lodge, Kerr confiscated it from her and looked through it, deciding in his wisdom that the contents exaggerated the extent of her mental health problems. Which of course, they did. The only possible way for people who need DLA to get it is to ham it up on the form: that's simply how it's done. But Kerr opted to destroy the form and complete a replacement in his own preferred style. Predictably, the reapplication failed, the woman's welfare benefits payments were withdrawn and she slid into dire poverty, worsening her mental distress. Kerr even had the audacity to threaten me when I moaned to his boss, Lisa Haywood, about this. He was bad news for the other staff and the clients at Homerton Friends Lodge, and he eventually met his death when Pete Shaughnessy threw him off a train moving at high speed on the way to a Mind annual conference in the year 2000.

Another controversy taking place towards the end of my stint running the advocacy service involved Dr Martin Deahl, the consultant psychiatrist for Brett Ward. With the apparent encouragement of his fellow doctors Trevor Turner and Martin Salter he invited a BBC film crew to film patients on his ward, to get footage for a documentary promoting community treatment orders as a beneficial way off extending psychiatrists' powers. The filming was controversial: most of the patients involved had been detained under sections of the Mental Health Act, begging the question that, if they were deemed incapable of consenting or otherwise to whatever treatment Deahl felt necessary, how could they have the capacity to consent to being shown on TV at their most vulnerable? And what would their neighbours think after they were discharged from hospital? We felt the patients were being exploited, and the Patients Council unsuccessfully called for Deahl's resignation, challenging his assertion that it was fine to lock up ten people who didn't really need sectioning if it prevented the one who really did need sectioning from getting away. Phil issued a press release suggesting that all psychiatrists should be locked up to prevent the occasional rogue from getting away, on the grounds that a Serbian shrink had recently committed atrocious war crimes in the war in the Balkans. Deahl survived; in fairness, I never found any real reasons to question his day to day clinical judgement.

Dumisa Morrison took over my job in Hackney after I left in January 1998. The job itself mutated into a more boundaried managerial position after I left, involving less hands-on work and a reduced presence at the hospital. The volunteers, feeling abandoned, all left and the project's profile declined. Hatice, the Turkish advocate, was frequently left on her own to deal with the advocacy needs of the whole hospital, regardless of their ethnicity. She'd always been a good advocate, but not so hot on the administrative side where she needed help. Now that such help was no longer forthcoming, paperwork fell behind and she was disciplined repeatedly by Dumisa. Stressed, unsupported and feeling bullied, she took sick leave and eventually resigned, diminishing the project further. The wages for my old post shot up rapidly while the client-load dropped. After a while Dumisa left to get another job where he was sacked after six months for bullying his staff. The advocacy project continued but in a much more conventionally professional, and arguably less effective way.

Fast forwarding a little, Dumisa turned up at a Mad Pride show in Camden in November 2002, and got talking to Shirley Pearson, a mental health advocate working in Southwark. They'd met at a black mental health workers network meeting. *"That's Robert Dellar"*, he observed, pointing at me, *"he used to be my boss.*

The whole time I worked with him, he was on drugs! He completely fucked himself up on drugs!"

Dumisa didn't realise that Shirley was a good friend of mine. I'd rarely touched illicit drugs during the time I'd worked with him: in fact, my poison then was strictly alcohol, and in spite of everything, nobody had been complaining about the quality or quantity of my work. I thought that his dismissal of me was something of a cheek, though it's true that people with bullying tendencies will always use people's vulnerabilities as a weapon against them. Part of the art of bullying is making people seem smaller and more wretched, to make the bully seem larger and more important by comparison. Dumisa must have felt insecure knowing that his work had been somewhat overshadowed by that of a scruffy, chaotic drunk.

By the time I left Hackney's advocacy department I'd split up with Sozen messily and hooked up with Tuba Karacalar, who on the whole was a good influence. Looking for new opportunities to cause trouble, I got a job as development worker for Southwark Mind, which needed to be set up from scratch.

Darling, Let's Have Another Baby

"*We really liked what you had to say and we're thinking about your suitability for the job*", Denise McKenna advised me over the phone, "*but we were worried that we could smell alcohol on your breath*".

At ten in the morning that day in December 1997, I'd been interviewed by Denise, who was a local user activist, as well as Fiona Hill, regional support worker for Mind groups across the south-east of England, and a couple of others whose names I had no cause ever to remember. Pete Shaughnessy was meant to have been one of the interviewers, but he'd been sectioned under the mental health act a few days previously and the hospital wouldn't let him out. Meeting him for the first time would have to wait for six weeks: a meeting which would lead to some of the most bizarre, radical and effective user activism ever seen, sending shock waves around the mental health field in this country and beyond.

I gave Denise some excuse or other, though the truth was that at the time I often started drinking before ten in the morning. Muffled voices were audible at the other end of the phone as the interview panel conferred. "*All right, the job's yours*" Denise said, not sounding completely convinced.

By this time, whether I liked it or not, I was increasingly finding myself classified as a 'user', though in fact my curriculum vitae of mental health service use went no further than counselling and anti-depressant tablets. Southwark Mind's executive committee had been turned into a user-led group in September 1997 when Denise and Pete carved up that year's annual general meeting. Prior to that, the committee had consisted of a motley crew of middle-class do-gooders, such as wives of consultant psychiatrists from the local hospital the Maudsley, and they would meet every two months or so to decide which worthy projects should be allocated the income received from a charity shop in East Dulwich, the posh part of Southwark. Effectively all that happened was that some of the Maudsley's work was subsidised. Pete and Denise changed this by persuading their mates to join Southwark Mind and voting themselves onto the committee, getting rid of the old guard. They now had their hands on the money which had accumulated in the bank account, and they decided to recruit someone to take Southwark Mind forward as a campaigning and creative grass-roots outfit. The job description was vague about how this should be done, which suited me by giving me plenty of room to manoeuvre and follow my own methods and ideas.

I arrived early and sober in Camberwell on January 29th 1998, and Denise was already in the small office at Cambridge House, a large building and charity in its own right running various projects, and renting rooms to smaller organisations. Pete wandered in soon after, announcing that he'd just come out of hospital and was depressed; nevertheless he quietly emitted a larger-than-life vibe. I'd heard of him already from Pete Fleischmann, who by now was working for Mental Health Media, a resource helping to improve user-led access to mainstream media. Fleischmann had told me about a highly intelligent and charismatic man he'd been working with, who he felt was capable of becoming a star user campaigner: of course, this turned out to be true. I'd also heard of Shaughnessy's pressure group, Reclaim Bedlam, which in 1997 had put the dampeners on ill-conceived '750th anniversary of Bedlam celebrations' organised by the local hospital. Pete had organised a demonstration against the celebrations at the Imperial War Museum, site of the original Bedlam, as well as pickets against various 'fun days' and feel-good events, attracting police surveillance. Pete knew that 750 years of torture, prejudice, boredom and incarceration were nothing to celebrate, and he was successful in taking this message to the media.

Dr Trevor Turner at the Homerton nut unit was notoriously sceptical about mental health service users' rights and activism.

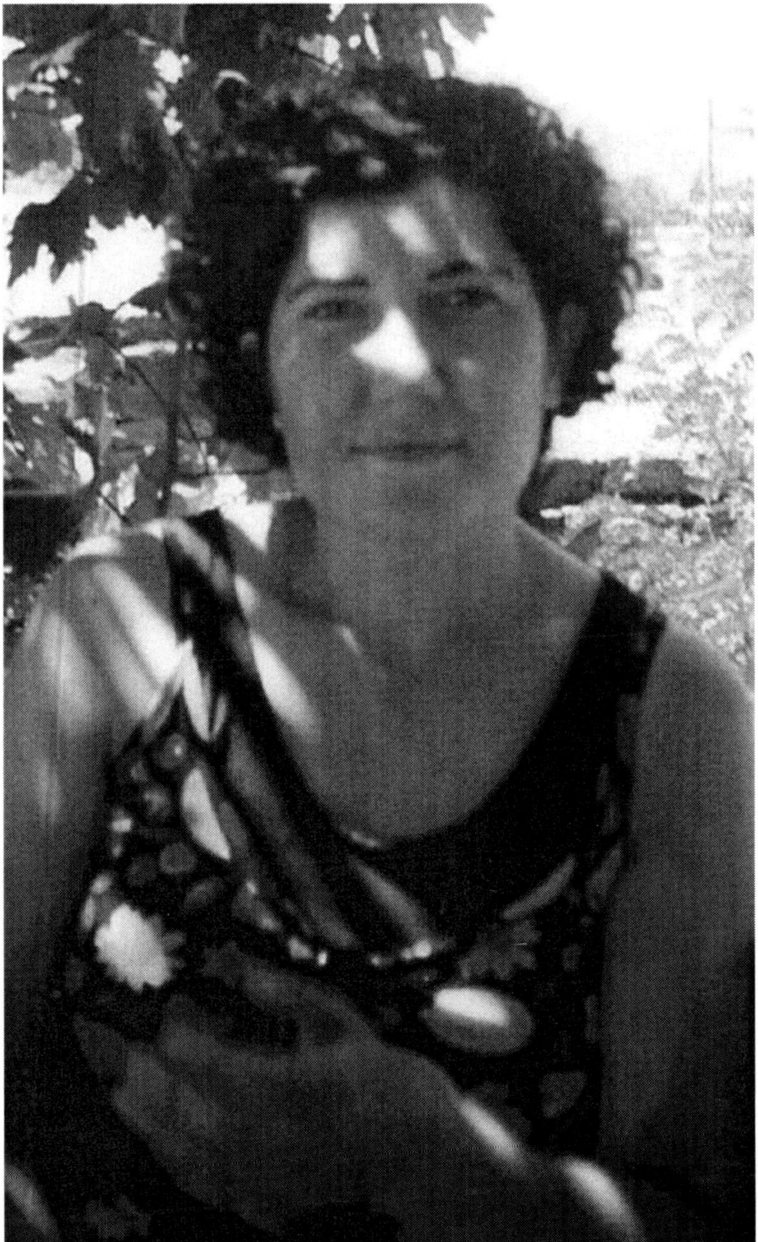

Tuba Karacalar

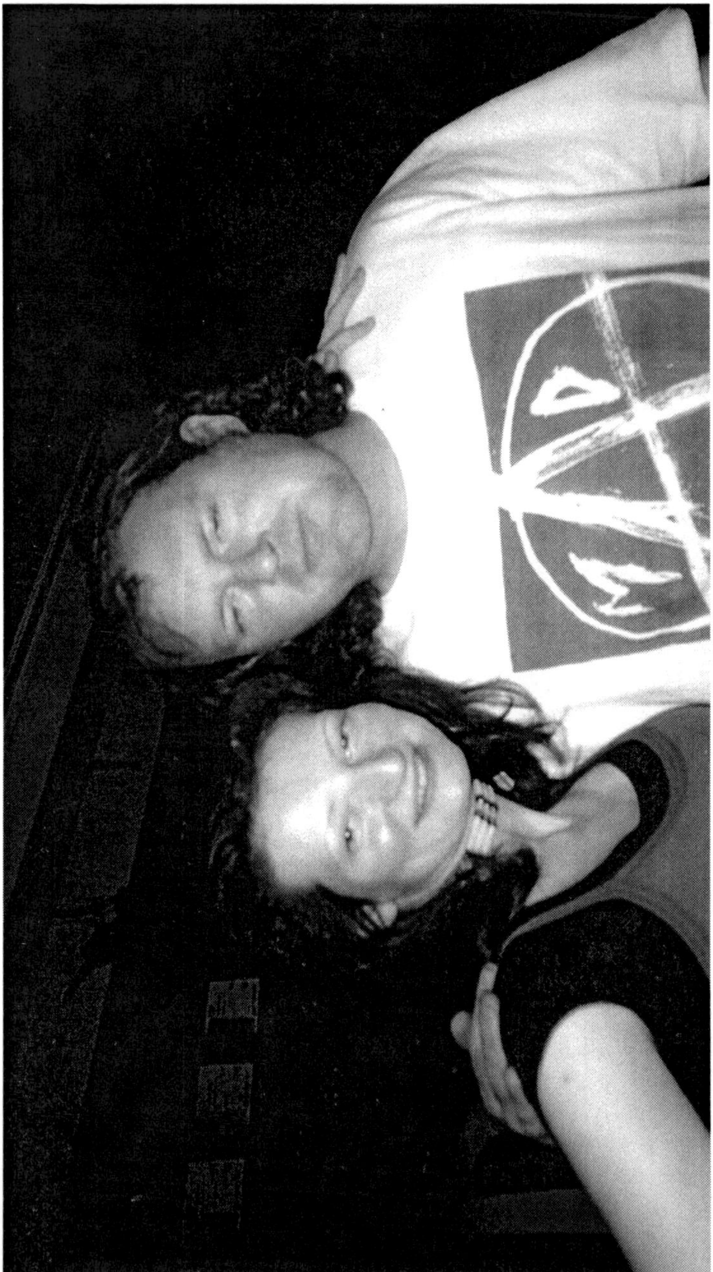

Rebecca Feines and Pete Shaughnessy, 20th June 1999.

He'd pinned a copy of Pete's press release advertising the demo on the door of his office as an ironic statement, as if to say: *"Look what these loonies are up to now, isn't it ridiculous!"* Turner had always had ambitions of hitting the media himself, believing himself to be an Anthony Clare in waiting, and took controversial right-wing positions on many mental health issues: counselling, for example, was a waste of time, catering only for the 'worried well', and therefore a waste of NHS resources which should be used only to treat people in acute psychotic crisis; and psychiatrists should be given the power to compulsorily medicate people in the community, just in case they became 'unwell'. Turner's ambitions were never fulfilled. Pete, on the other hand, whose hilarious, polemical press release had made perfect sense to me, went on to achieve fame.

Like most people, I warmed to Pete immediately. Pete and Denise took me that day to the Lorrimore, a local mental health day centre which had open access, not requiring referrals from social workers or other professionals, and which therefore had a less institutional feel than some such places; I was introduced to the staff and some of the punters. There had been an informal agreement between the Lorrimore and Southwark Mind that the new worker, who turned out to be me, would help staff their monthly Saturday night disco. I immediately rejected this idea, pointing out that it amounted to a potential conflict of interests, as well as a redirection of Southwark Mind's resources into mainstream service provision, which I didn't think was meant to be the idea. When I did make it to their disco on one occasion, simply to get to know a few local users, it was late in the evening and I was stumbling about a little after a few cans, which apparently didn't pass without comment. After leaving the Lorrimore on my first day at work, I was taken to Mary's caff in Camberwell Road, which would become one of my haunts, and at times a reserve office space for the next five years.

I had to think carefully about how to get Southwark Mind up and running. My job had been advertised partly on the back of a funding application submitted to the National Lotteries Board by the then-treasurer Alan Mepstead. The management committee had assumed it was a fait accompli that the bid would be successful, but a few days after I started the work a letter arrived turning it down, so my first task was to raise the money for my own wages and running costs. I managed to do this quite quickly thanks to the City Parochial Foundation. Denise, Pete and Myself also managed to chuck together the first issue of *Southwark Mind Newsletter,* released in March 1998. 400 copies were posted to Mind members or left lying around day centres and hospitals: the magazine went on to be prolific and very popular. Drawing on my experience of editing fanzines, I used a punk-style cut and paste technique resembling *Sniffin' Glue, Vague, Ripped and Torn* and other classic zines from the late 1970s, and I clung stubbornly to this format right up until issue 61 five years later, after which the editorship passed temporarily to Danielle Rosier. Most local charities' magazines and newssheets were over-mediated by computer technology, and looked as if they contained the minutes of a board meeting: boring, and useful only to satisfy funders. The punk approach gave the rag a human, down-at-heel touch which was charming and set it aside from its peers, resonating with mental health service users in South London as well as other people. The humorous, lucid, often scandalous tabloid-style articles written by Pete Shaughnessy and myself helped it become a hit, and for punters it was often the only item of mail to arrive each month that wasn't a bill or a pizza delivery advert. People enjoyed its flippancy and sense of rebellion, and this showed that mental health didn't always have to be a morbid, serious subject, a suggestion which at that point, oddly, had rarely been made.

The next book I put out made *Southwark Mind Newsletter* look like the *Daily Mail. Seaton Point* was the result of the writing group I'd set up two years previously. It was ostensibly written by Martin, Ted, Mally, Lucy, Emma, Rob and myself, though in fact me, Ted and Martin wrote most of it with the others simply having cameo slots.

It was a miracle that this novel was ever completed, let alone published, given the state the lot of us were in at the time. Most of us were battling with varying degrees of alcoholism as well as dealing with nervous breakdowns, traumatic relationship endings or homelessness. I had to rewrite many of the other authors' parts, as some of the writers literally lost the plot and the text became disjointed. By the time that it was published a further draft would have helped, but by then I was getting sick of working on it and simply wanted to get the fucker out. A sordid tale of anarchism, alcoholism and gratuitous sex scenes, it's set in Seaton Point, a real-life 21-storey tower block in the Nightingale

Southwark Mind MANIFESTO

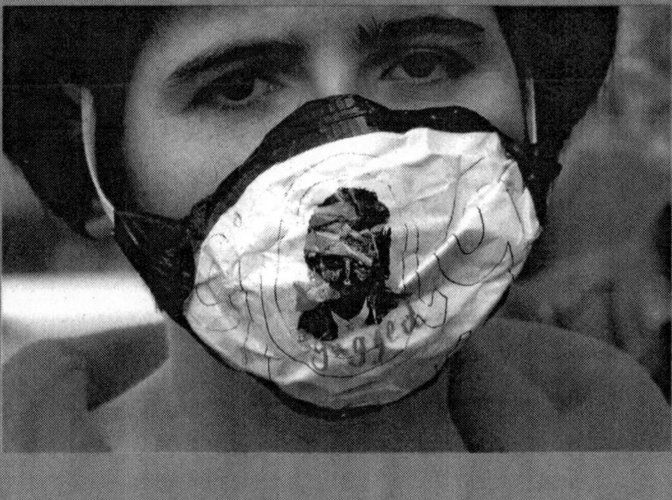

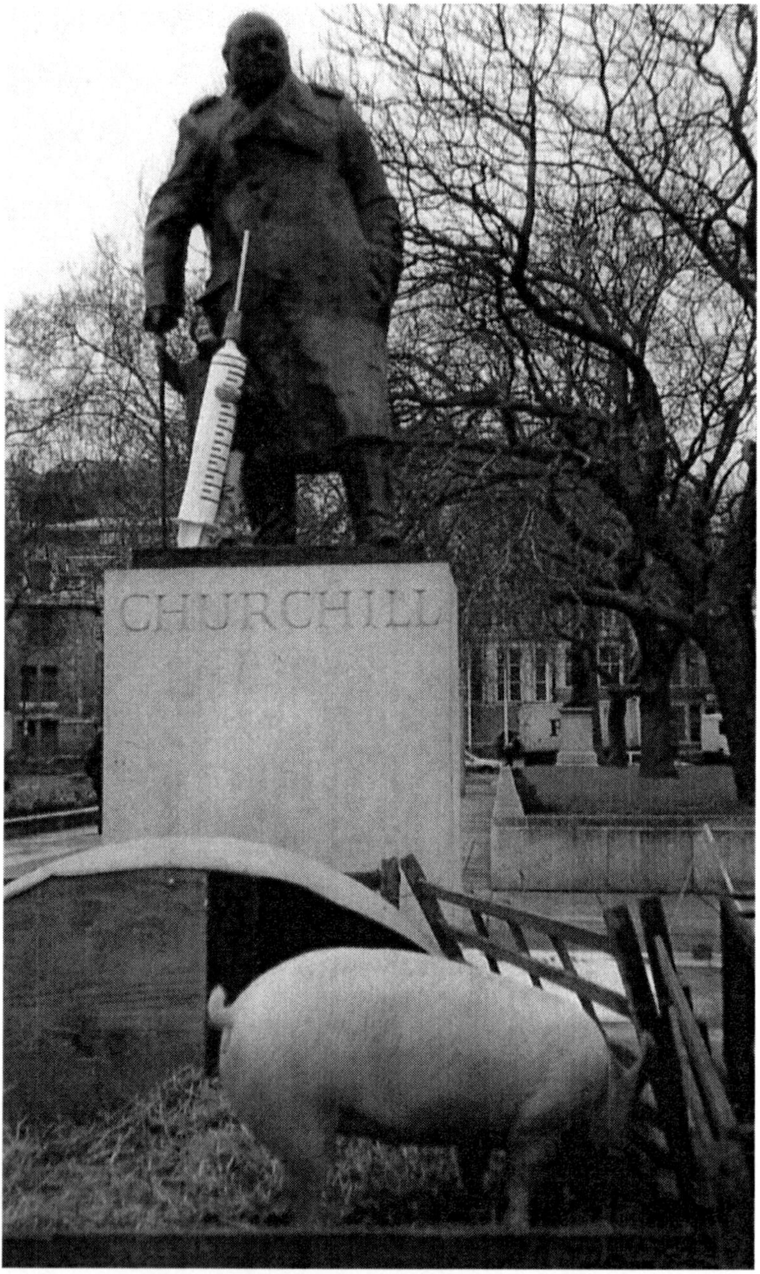

Lynne Clayton with the Mad Pride syringe

sink estate in Lower Clapton, Hackney, where both Jon Active and Ted Curtis live. The book is confusing and contains far too many characters, but bizarrely has ended up on the curricula of English literature university courses, some boffins apparently having decided that it's an example of the 'modern gothic' English novel.

The book's launch party was held one evening at Chat's Palace, which in the novel itself was burnt to the ground with Jon Active inside as part of an occult ritual. The show featured a one-off reunion performance from Martin's 1980s pop-punk trio Salad From Atlantis, sets from the Astronauts and avant-garde saxophonist Lol Coxhill, and readings by most of the authors. I was drunk but coherent on stage, but Ted was more drunk than I was. In fact, he was paralytic, having imbibed around fifteen cans of Tennents Super during the day. He had to be helped onto the stage, with somebody stationed next to his seat to help make sure he didn't injure himself when he fell off, and another person had to hold the book open for him at the right pages because unaided he kept dropping it. Drunkenly he slurred a few words here and there, forgot what he was doing, fell asleep, woke up again when prodded, and slurred a few more words from a different part of the book, resulting in a variation of the cut-up technique. For most audience members Ted was the star of the show, and it was an appropriate summary of the book's content matter as well as the state most of us had been in when it was written. I can't even remember exactly which parts I wrote and which were by the other people.

In the audience was Ben Watson, a well-spoken SWP member who was shacked up with party comrade Esther Leslie, who I'd known years back at Sussex University. I'd met Ben a couple of times before at mutual friend Stewart Home's book launches, and my initial impressions had been misleading. He'd criticised my punk anthology *Gobbing, Pogoing and Gratuitous Bad Language* for not being avant-garde enough to portray punk authentically; I'd simply thought *"who's this posh cunt?"* Ben and Esther are both Marxist academics, and since our initial meetings I'd read Ben's masterpiece *Art, Class and Cleavage*, which is a hugely complex, funny and erudite philosophical tract which probably would have had him kicked out of the SWP had his party comrades been able to understand a word of it. Terry Eagleton, who didn't like the book, described it as being from *"the surrealist wing of the So-*

cialist Workers Party, who could probably hold their meetings in a phone box". I congratulated him on his achievement; he told me he'd liked *Seaton Point*. I altered my opinion of the bastard and we became friends.

Meanwhile, Southwark Mind was kicking off. Jolie Goodman and Lynne Clayton came on board as management committee members and both would prove invaluable. As a method of launching the new charity and helping to determine its future direction, we set up a conference to carve out the way forward for the user movement in Southwark, posing questions concerning whether we wanted to continue trying to influence mental health services planning and policy by turning up at professional meetings of bureaucrats and arguing the toss. This tactic had been tried and, for the most part, failed over the previous few years, undermined by lack of support, structure and supervision for user representatives; lack of a demonstrable constituency, leaving representatives open to often justifiable complaints that they spoke only for themselves, and that their views conflicted with those of 'ordinary' users who wouldn't have dreamt of bothering to go to meetings; and representatives' frequent inability to master professional jargon, employed by services managers and commissioners as a way of making their work incomprehensible to the public, shrouding it in secrecy. Also, it was intimidating for a lone user who bought their clothes at charity shops, hadn't had a bath or a shave in two weeks and chain-smoked roll-ups created from dog-ends scavenged from the pavement, to be surrounded by suits who smoked only the most expensive cigars and who had been to Oxford University. We wondered whether we could influence policy using other means.

Sixty or so local users attended the conference, which took place upstairs at the Lorrimore in July 1998. Workshops were held on various pertinent issues: Arun Mushiana led one on ethnicity and user-led mental health issues; Cath Collins, chair of the similarly user-led Lambeth Mind, ran one with Denise beginning with the premise that 'we are the experts on our own distress', and there were two others. Panel discussions took place with Pete Fleischmann, Fiona Hill and others on the panel. The conference resolved to boycott the suits' meetings and instead hold our own, inviting professionals along to negotiate with them on our own terms, in our own language and setting our own agendas.

Following the business covered by the conference we laid out a feast in the day centre downstairs, which in truth was all that had attracted many of the participants along, and there was a music set from the Astronauts which went down well in spite of a faulty sound system. I was left with some thinking to do. After a while and some informal discussions with Pete, Denise and others, I hit on the idea of setting up Southwark User Council, which I envisaged as comprising elected representatives of various day centres, hospital wards and independent user groups who would form a committee. The vision was that these reps would take away agenda items, discuss them with their fellow users at their specific locations, discover the consensus or perhaps range of opinions, then bring these back, monitored and demonstrable to the monthly meeting, to which select suits would be invited. The advantages would be manifold. Operating under what was by then becoming an efficient corporate user group umbrella, the reps would have somewhere to go for effective support, guidance and supervision. Consulting other users in their groups and monitoring the responses would undermine bureaucratic claims that the opinions put forward were unrepresentative. The reps would be paid to the limit of what they could earn without their welfare benefits being compromised, which at the time was fifteen pounds a week for those on incapacity benefit. And potentially they could present a united front in a forum in which users would have control over the proceedings and, in theory at least, call the shots. To their credit, the suits from the Health Authority and local Social Services all thought this was a constructive idea, particularly because it would help them fulfil their statutory targets regarding user consultation which increasingly were becoming a legal obligation. First, I needed to tout this plan around the various user groups, day centres and hospitals, to whip up grass-roots interest and fine-tune the mechanics.

While this was happening, the six-month probationary period for my job ended. I had an external supervisor, Rick Henderson, who ran the Independent Advocacy Service in Camberwell and in his youth had fronted an anarcho-punk band. Prior to meeting with Rick for my probationary assessment where my work performance would be discussed, Pete warned me that whispers of alcohol being frequently on my breath would be raised as an issue. Denise, herself a recovering alcoholic, had raised her suspicions with Rick, and Pete, with reservations, had backed them up. This warning came during a meeting in the pub, after which I had to put Pete in a taxi home and point the driver in the right direction. Forewarned, I pre-empted Rick's queries, putting him on the back foot, and got away with it – presumably because my work was perceived as being fine, and because a buzz was beginning to form around Southwark Mind which nobody involved really wished to jeopardise.

Nevertheless, the incident gave me a jolt, and as it wasn't my intention to let my problems threaten my work, I booked myself into the community alcohol team in Haringey to arrange a supervised detoxification. I'd never thought about getting a GP in Hackney after I'd moved, so as far as primary health services were aware I still lived in Tottenham. If I'd tried to stop drinking without help at this point, I would have had severe DTs making me incapable of getting much done for a few days, and the pressure of my workload made this appear to me to be inadvisable. In fact, the alcohol team demanded that I took two weeks off during the detox, so I lied to them and pretended not to be going into work. Medically supervised, 'ambulatory' as opposed to inpatient detoxifications involve turning up at the crack of dawn every morning for a week or so to pick up industrial quantities of benzodiazepines or similar – in this case Librium – to help ease the withdrawal symptoms. After a week I was clean. I then began to see an alcohol counsellor in Hackney, a trainee who was pleasant but not skilled enough to be of any real use. My first ever spell of true adult sobriety lasted for ten weeks, until Boxing Day. I'd split up with Tuba and, briefly and ill-advisedly, hooked up with Mina again, spending Christmas day with her family, within which there were some disturbing dynamics leading them to engage in a heartbreaking display of charades and collective denial. Upset by this, I used it as an excuse to relapse the next day, setting off another binge which lasted for six months. If I hadn't had this excuse, I'd have found another soon enough, although I was too naive at the time to be fully aware of this.

This six month period was nevertheless an intense and inspired time. I fed from the energy of Southwark Mind colleagues, in particular Pete Shaughnessy, and wanted to be at the heart of reaching for new collective heights for the user movement and its attendant campaigning.

A lot happened in a very short space of time. The New Labour government was then, in early 1999, preparing to rewrite the 1983 Mental Health Act, giving massively increased powers to psychiatrists and the pharmaceutical industry. Community treatment orders were promised, enabling doctors to force their patients in the community to take psychiatric medication against their will, under threat of being removed to hospital if they failed to comply. The previous situation was that only hospital in-patients could be coerced in this manner, and even then not if they were voluntary patients but only if they were detained under a section of the Mental Health Act. Remember, these drugs may have numbed some of the symptoms of psychosis, but none of the causes, and only at the expense of numbing the entirety of the patients' experiences and causing severe, life-shortening physical ill health: not for nothing were these drugs known as the 'liquid cosh'. Many service users didn't fancy being given Parkinson's disease.

The perniciousness and horror of community treatment orders cannot be understated. Pharmaceutical manufacturers such as Glaxo and Novartis had been using a variety of means, both directly and by proxy, to lobby the medical profession and the government for years for the extension of compulsory treatment powers into people's homes, knowing that if more people were forced to take their drugs their profits would increase. The pharmaceutical industry, second only to the arms industry, is the most powerful, secretive and corrupt business sector in the world. It systematically falsifies the research it conducts into its own drugs, and routinely lobbies the medical profession to invent new 'illnesses' to be treated by newly developed medications. Frequently, new drugs are developed prior to the inventions of the illnesses they are supposed to treat. Consequently the list of psychiatric symptoms and diagnoses has increased exponentially, year after year, since the first psychiatric drugs were invented in the 1950s. The mental health sector is far more susceptible to such manipulations and deceit than physical health, because of the unscientific and conjectural nature of mental health diagnosis and treatment, a situation exploited mercilessly by drug companies.

Drug companies pay doctors to have their names attached to articles published in health journals, articles which in fact have been written by the companies' advertising agencies in order to give credence to the largely bogus research statistics and optimistic claims promoting their products. They hand out mountains of freebies to doctors, hospitals and GPs' surgeries which themselves could be worth enough annually to wipe out the national debt of a third world country or two. In 1999, everywhere you went there were yellow Lustral mugs featuring smiley happy faces, Prozac post-it notes, calendars, biros, pocket calculators and mouse-pads, while psychiatrists were constantly being invited to trade conferences which doubled as drug launches, where the shrinks were plied to prescribe the latest wonder-drug with vast banquets, accommodation in five-star hotels, sexual favours and cocaine. I'm not saying that there is never any point in taking psychiatric medication. I've tried anti-depressants myself, though probably during those times I was drinking too much to be aware of any effect. I am saying that we should be aware and beware of the corporate interests lurking behind these so-called cures, interests which unscrupulously put profits before people. Coercing people to take drugs is more of an economic imperative than a health issue, and the often-promoted idea that this in any way prevents violent crime is nothing more than an obscene corporate smokescreen.

The medical profession and pharmaceutical industry have never, however, lobbied for the creation of legal powers compelling people to take drugs marketed as relieving depression. They know that such an idea would be a non-starter, because depression only publicly affects those experiencing it and those closest to them: depressed people are not on the whole considered to be a nuisance to society at large, except as a burden on the welfare state. Community treatment orders are designed only to control psychosis, which is sometimes more extroverted, and therefore more public and noticeable. When Frank Dobson, who was health secretary when this bill was being drafted, called 'mentally ill' people 'nuisance neighbours', he was referring not to those of us susceptible to depression, 6000 of whom kill themselves each year in Britain alone, according to official statistics which overlook the very many suicides which have not been recorded as such. He was referring to people with diagnoses of schizophrenia, manic-depression or bipolar disorder as it has been re-branded, or personality disorders: people responsible for the very occasional homicide or act of violence which can be attributed, often falsely, to their conditions, and which usually take place – as is the case with 'sane' people – when the offender is drunk. For drug companies to widen their markets, they need

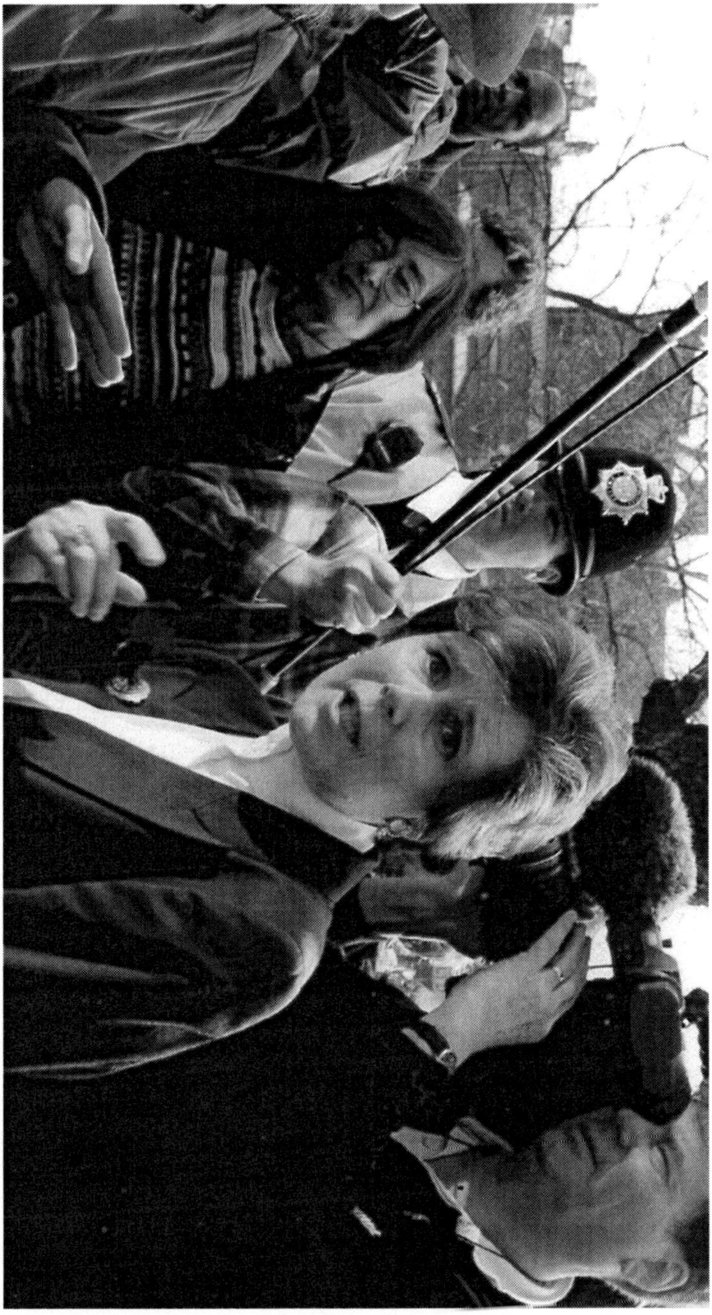

SANE Chief Exec Marjorie Wallace being hassled outside her Whitechapel Offices at the Reclaim Bedlam demo, 15th March 1999

to manufacture public belief that coerced drugging has a public benefit which is wider than the patient's own good.

Statistically, the rate of homicide and violent crime by people with psychotic diagnoses is about the same as the rate for the 'sane'. But mad people are picked on. Politicians are rarely concerned with the treatment of people at risk to themselves. It's easier for them to target those who go against the grain enough to be deemed psychotic, worthy of being suppressed and silenced, and who offend the prejudices and sensibilities of middle England dwellers whose votes are coveted.

Drug companies fund much of the work taking place at the Royal College of Psychiatry, courting medical acquiescence with their marketing ploys, buying influence. To be fair, large numbers of people within the psychiatric profession have opposed this situation, although this only really became apparent towards the very end of the nineties. The drug companies also fund some charities to do their campaigning, and therefore marketing for them, influencing parliament and public opinion.

Early in 1999, chief among these charities were SANE, an acronym for 'Schizophrenia – A National Emergency', and the Zito Trust. The latter group was set up by Jayne Zito, whose husband Michael had been murdered a few years previously by Chris Clunis: stabbed in the eye at Finsbury Park tube station. Clunis, later sent to Broadmoor, had a diagnosis of schizophrenia and had fallen between gaps in services owing to peripatetic behaviour. Understandably distraught, Jayne Zito had set up her own charity, which campaigned to restrict the civil liberties of psychiatric service users in the mistaken belief that this would help prevent such tragedies taking place in the future. A media spokesman, Michael Howlett, was recruited, and his public pronouncements seemed designed to set public mental health awareness back decades. The charity consisted only of Howlett and Jayne Zito, but the pair had a disproportionately vocal impact on the media and the government, helped by the fact that Jayne lived in Frank Dobson's constituency in Camden, attending several of his surgeries and urging changes in the law to allow mental health patients effectively to be shackled. Dobson picked up on these demands and a battle around community treatment orders becoming law kicked off, with resistance from the user movement. Jayne Zito's actions were doubtlessly well-intentioned and heartfelt, but they were wrong. She was rumoured to have had an affair with the producer of the TV programme *Panorama*, which consequently or otherwise ran a show highlighting the 'danger' of those mad people not locked safely away in institutions.

The actions of SANE were altogether more difficult to fathom. The charity's founder and chief executive, Marjorie Wallace, was a journalist with inside knowledge of media manipulation, and an interest in mental health apparently sparked off by issues within her family. Heavily funded by drug companies, SANE prolifically pushed the media message that psychiatric patients are violent and should be locked up. SANE became perceived to be a credible group, in part because they spent a disproportionate amount of their income on advertising campaigns which made them look a bigger concern than they really were. In fact, their only 'service' was a telephone helpline giving advice to mad people's relatives, from a mainstream medical perspective.

SANE's first major campaign was an onslaught of billboard posters, featuring the face of a woman looking distressed, with the strap-line: *"You don't have to be mentally ill to suffer from mental illness"*. What they meant by this was that it's not only the 'mentally ill' who are distressed with their conditions, but also the people around them who are forced to put up with their existence. The poster drew a lot of criticism, and after many years was replaced by an almost identical one with the slogan changed to *"you don't have to be mentally ill to experience mental illness"*, a slightly softer way of saying the same thing, and promoting the same discrimination.

I'd subverted the poster whilst working in Hackney, replacing the face with that of the then Tory health secretary Virginia Bottomley, cutting her eyes out of the picture then replacing them upside down, making her look really evil, a tactic I'd borrowed from Crass. Using the same lettering as the original poster, I wrote: *"You don't have to be mad to be mentally ill, but it helps"*. The altered poster circulated widely, and many people thought it was authentic SANE material.

It's hard to estimate how great a part our march on SANE played in escalating the struggle for mental health service users' rights. Nothing like this had ever happened before. Survivors Speak Out had once attempted to demonstrate outside SANE's offices but it had only amounted to a small picket, which was dispersed after the charity called the old bill. The 1999 march on SANE was officially organised by Reclaim Bedlam, though in

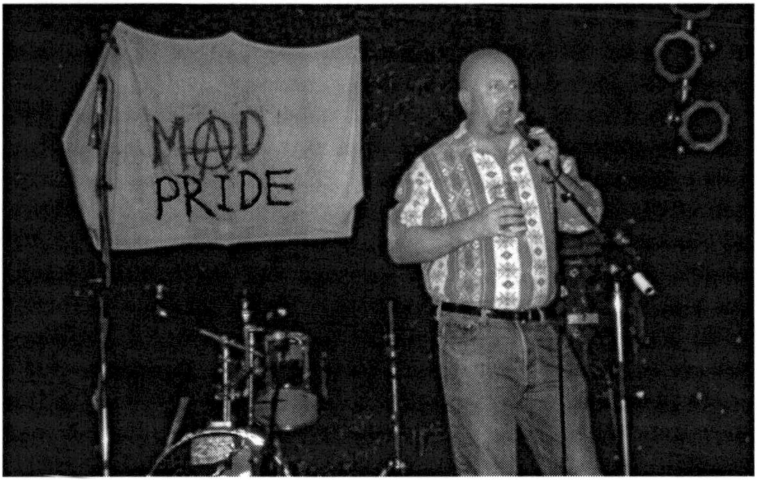

Simon Barnett

fact Southwark Mind provided the finance and nerve centre, and the event took user radicalism to a hitherto unprecedented level. Southwark Mind couldn't officially take responsibility for this demonstration for fear of trouble with the charities commission. SANE spent a lot of time trying to find out who was behind the action in advance of it and suspected Pete of being involved, initially issuing a press release claiming that it was being organised by another of his projects, the Bermondsey and Rotherhithe Mental Health Support Group, which was a self-help group not directly involved with campaigning. SANE's press release anticipated *"a handful of people from South East London"*.

Southwark Mind was almost alone amongst London user groups in not being telephoned or threatened in the run-up to the event. I was something of a grey eminence at the time, a little like Stalin prior to becoming the dictator of Russia. Many detailed planning meetings took place, most of them in the pub, though we also found a new home: Pumpkins, a top, cheap vegetarian caff in Clarence Road, Hackney, subsequently called Pogo's and a regular supplier of catering for anarchist book fairs and similar events.

We were demonstrating against the proposed community treatment orders and held SANE, in part, responsible for the threat due to their role in whipping up media hatred of mental health service users, with Marjorie Wallace repeatedly drawing a link between 'mad' and 'dangerous' in her articles and through her status as a spokesperson. Phil Murphy, mindful of the fact that the health secretary, by now Paul Boateng, had denied that community treatment orders would involve punters being *"forcibly medicated over their kitchen tables"*, had the idea of putting a kitchen table outside SANE's headquarters and staging mock forced injections with a giant syringe. The group agreed that this was a fine idea and commissioned the Hackney-based sculptor Cat Monstersmith to build the syringe, which was seven feet long and looked great.

The survivor movement was evolving as a result of the planning of the demo, and it was looking further into the future. Pete introduced me to Simon Barnett and Mark Roberts, who by then were the rump of Survivors Speak Out which was on its last legs. The original movers and shakers behind this group had gone on to get careers as trainers, researchers, consultants and after-dinner speakers, and good luck to them all. Peter Campbell, David Crepaz-Keays, Jan Wallcraft, Jim Read and others were spending their time educating and negotiating with professionals from user perspectives, and making an income by trotting out their stories and often changeable opinions at conferences and training events. They'd outgrown their initial, pioneering work and were reaping the personal benefits of it, as they had every right to do, Survivors Speak Out having outlived its use. Simon and Mark were trying to keep the show on the road, but also tentatively looking in other directions. We met in Pumpkins and they told me and Pete about an idea they'd been carrying around in their heads for two years, but hadn't yet the skills and confidence to put into practice. The pair had attended a Gay Pride festival in Finsbury Park and concluded: why not Mad Pride? Simon described his vision of putting on low-key pub gigs, featuring punk musicians and others promoting the cause. Pete and I supported this idea but thought that it could be more ambitious.

Meanwhile, we mailed every user group in Britain we knew about – in other words nearly all of them – advertising the demo. We invested in numerous props, not only the syringe but also drums, whistles, banners, party hooters, white doctors' coats with slogans on the back, t-shirts reading *"schizo and proud"*, plastic toy swords from Woolworths, tridents – because we're the devil – and a megaphone. Cath Collins liaised with the police to get the okay for the demo before SANE could pester them. We were taking this seriously.

SANE were having kittens, issuing hasty, ill-considered media statements shooting themselves in the foot, and still frantically trying and failing to identify the ringleaders so that they could intimidate us. Pete Fleischmann from Mental Health Media helped us compose our own more successful press releases, and we described Marjorie Wallace as being to mental health what Enoch Powell was to race relations. SANE responded with a press release appearing to defend Enoch Powell, stating correctly but ill-advisedly that he'd been the architect of the care in the community policy during his stint as Tory health secretary in the early sixties, making it look as if SANE were fans of his. Additionally, challenged by the media about our perfectly true claims that SANE ignored user perspectives, Wallace claimed that she routinely consulted several user groups. Asked to name some, she struggled to remember two she'd heard of: Communicate, who at the time were the Patients' Council at the Maudsley hospital in Camberwell, and UKAN, short for the United Kingdom Advocacy Network, then a Sheffield-based umbrella organisation for user groups nationwide. The media approached these groups, who confirmed that Wallace was lying and that neither she nor SANE had ever had any contact at all with them, although UKAN's boss Terry Simpson was quoted in the *Big Issue* as saying that he was looking forward to attending the demo.

Pete and myself decided to visit SANE's offices on reconnaissance, to demand – as was our legal entitlement – a copy of their annual report and accounts. The intimidated suits drew a collective sharp intake of breath as we wandered around the building being nosey, and they had no choice but to hand us a copy, showing that enough of their income came from pharmaceutical companies to suggest that SANE's media forays were little more than a front for them. Wallace at the time wrote a regular column for the *Daily Mail*, and a recent one had the headline *"VICTORY!"* referring to the government's recent decision to draft a bill to enforce community treatment orders. Photocopies of the column were plastered all over the walls and notice boards of SANE's gaff, a fact which made Wallace's later protestations that SANE had never agreed with the idea even more laughable.

Dieter Cole, Debbie McNamara and myself went flyposting at night to generate more publicity for the demo which was sched-

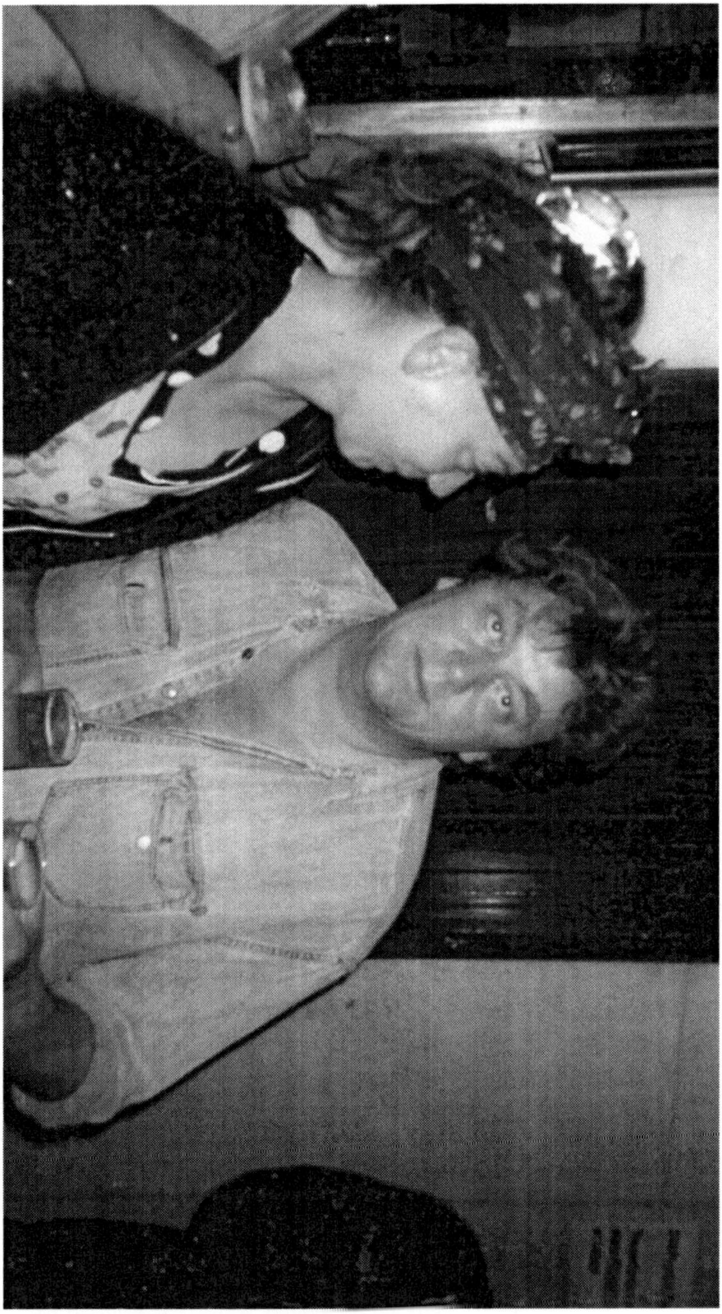

Cat Monstersmith and Jackie Leven

uled for March 15th 1999. We stuck large posters everywhere, some bearing the slogan *"Beware the Ides of March, Wallace"* beside a picture of her looking evil: at bus stops, on the doors of day centres, over billboards and disused shops, and most satisfyingly, dozens of them on the walls of SANE's own building in Whitechapel, which would have amused the staff when they arrived for work the following morning. Another flyposting expedition was more stressful, when two of us were caught red-handed in Stoke Newington by the old bill. Two young coppers explained that if we'd been Turkish people putting up 'Free Ocalan' posters, they would have charged us with criminal damage and being drunk and disorderly. Ocalan was the leader of a Kurdish nationalist militia who'd recently been captured by the Turkish police, and because of Hackney's ethnic demographics this was something of a local issue; the cops clearly didn't distinguish between Turkish and Kurdish. However, because we were white, they told us, they were prepared to let us go.

Another depressing incident in the lead-up to the demo involved my old employers City and Hackney Mind. Debbie McNamara and Earil Hunter had been leafleting Hackney conscientiously, advertising the event, and went to Homerton Friends Lodge, still managed by Len Kerr who by then had yet to meet his tragic demise at Pete Shaughnessy's murderous hands. Kerr confiscated the leaflets the pair had tried to distribute, and frogmarched them out of the premises. Earil must have been remarkably self-restrained, as he could easily have battered the fuck out of the manager had he felt so inclined. We wondered who the hell this Kerr character thought he was, censoring information. Didn't his clients have every right to make up their own minds regarding the rights and wrongs of the demo? In his opinion apparently not. Was he trying to turn the place into a patriarchal, patronising institution? Perhaps he was.

Roger Harris, the excellent local Mind director during my stint there, had left to get a commissioning job in Haringey which paid better. He'd been replaced by Lisa Haywood, the pioneer user activist who in my time with Hackney Mind had been a very good advice co-ordinator: she was good-humoured, broad-minded and committed, and I'd got on well with her. Promotion may have altered her priorities. Certainly her clothes and haircut became more conventionally professional; perhaps her attitude had too.

Debbie phoned Lisa to complain about her treatment by the doomed day centre manager. Lisa defended him as well as SANE, correctly pointing out that Marjorie Wallace alone couldn't alone be held responsible for the threat of community treatment orders, and in fact we'd never claimed that this had been the case. Debbie must have stated her point of view assertively, and Lisa wrote her a letter complaining about her *"abusive and threatening"* phone call as well as raising the issue with the City and Hackney Mind executive committee which, only having heard one side of the story, concurred with Lisa and censured Debbie. Around the same time Hackney Patients Council, which still employed Debbie, was banished from Mind's Tudor Road offices, though the two incidents were not necessarily related. Lisa claimed to have a witness to the 'abusive' phone call: Maya Wadhwani, Alison Bugg's replacement as admin co-ordinator. Maya's recollection differed significantly from Lisa's. She claimed to feel too intimidated and professionally compromised to publicly challenge Lisa's version of events, and rang Debbie at home to tell her she didn't think she'd been in any way been at fault. I was disappointed with Lisa, whose stance in this dispute seemed out of character. Debbie received a nasty letter from the executive committee. I wrote to them defending her, and received a letter back which was dismissive.

The sickest thing about this was that, at the very same time, Debbie had taken the lead in organising the Hackney end of City and Hackney Mind staff member Jo Crane's funeral arrangements.

Jo, who I'd met when she was a patient at the Junction day ward at the old Hackney Hospital, had been a great source of help for the advocacy project and the Patients Council, and had eventually got a paid, fixed-contract job with Hackney Mind as a research expert. Shortly after her term ended, she threw herself from the infamous 'Suicide Bridge' in Archway onto a busy dual carriageway, dying six or seven hours later. Debbie organised all the transport from Hackney to the funeral in Berkshire, and did all of the necessary phoning around informing people, including the rest of Hackney Mind's staff, of the terrible news.

Jo had been a good friend to me and to the rest of the Hackney crew. Highly intelligent, caring and witty, she'd spent much of the previous few years in hospital, often in the slammer – the so-called Bevan Ward – where she was always the only female patient in a locked pressure cooker environment with seventeen young men. Jo was also the only person on the ward with a diagnosis of depression, rather than a 'psychotic illness' like schizophrenia or manic-depression. To put it very mildly, this was not a therapeutic environment for her.

Even in hospital and at her most unwell, Jo would always be concerned about how me and her other crazy friends were, and acted more worried about this than about herself when we visited her on Bevan Ward. One of the kindest and most depressed people I've met in my life, she still found the resources and energy not to let go of this caring. When she was on open wards and allowed to go out occasionally, it would provide me with a good excuse to go to the pub where we'd while away work time playing pool: despite the fact that she was a recovering alcoholic, she always maintained a passion for the game and was happy to spend time in bars. I'd been to visit her on Bevan Ward on the way to the famous Hackney Anarchy Week launch party starring Alternative TV, and was already so drunk it was a miracle that they let me into the ward. I sat there smoking with her, verbally insulting and patronising the young trainee nurses keeping her within touching distance under 'close observation', and I got away with it. This is a happy memory. Jo also starred in a posthumously screened BBC2 television documentary about living with depression, in which she describes the experience eloquently and charismatically whilst swimming with dolphins in the Irish Sea.

Jo's suicide followed a string of comparable tragedies, including three friends' brothers dying in a period of one month. Phil Murphy's brother had thrown himself from the top of a tower block in Israel during the time that Phil was living with me. Mina's brother Sasha, who for some months had lived with us in Tottenham, had successfully gassed himself in a car at the second attempt. Nikki Sudden's brother Epic Soundtracks, the drummer in the pair's 1970s band Swell Maps, appeared to have overdosed on prescription medication. It was bewildering. Hundreds of people turned up at Jo's funeral in Berkshire, many of the Hackney folks getting there in a nutter bus driven by Julie Hathaway. It was heartbreaking.

Holidays in the Sun

The day of the SANE demo arrived and three hundred raving lunatics congregated outside the Royal London Hospital for the short march along Whitechapel High Street to SANE's nerve centre, which was opposite a small park for street drinkers. SANE didn't know what the fuck had hit them: they'd been prepared only for a small picket. With the noise generated by whistles, chants, screams, whooping and drumming, our numbers seemed larger than they actually were and we scared the shit out of the staff peering nervously from the first floor windows as we piled into the park. We whipped out our kitchen table and giant syringe, supplemented by a large box of cornflakes and a carton of milk, and demonstrators disguised as medical staff in white coats administered mock injections over the table to a succession of victims, providing ample photo opportunities for the media, who were out in force.

As we stood around gloating, Marjorie Wallace bravely came out of her headquarters and faced us. "*We've never supported community treatment orders*" she lied, when in fact her campaigning had been partly responsible for the threat of them in the first place. Wallace's new take was that people defaulting on medication should simply be 'removed' to a 'clinical setting', which could be loosely defined as anywhere from a hospital to a police station, where they could be kept until it was felt safe that they'd resume taking their drugs obediently. Exactly how people should be 'removed' to these safe settings was never made clear, but it seemed that our demo had persuaded SANE to make this minor policy change.

We gave the chief executive a suitably hard time, and it was an enlivening and morale-boosting occasion as protesters shouted "*fuck off, Wallace!*" and "*go back to your nice office, we don't like you!*" at her face in front of the TV cameras. After a while the old bill insisted on leading her back to her building for her own safety. Humiliated, she was swallowed up by her plush offices. People were floating around the small park with pictures of Wallace impaled on their tridents; some of these pictures were burnt on the doorstep of SANE's headquarters. It was a spectacular performance. Frank Bangay bellowed one of his poems, 'That Old Taboo', over the megaphone whilst staring and gesticulating wildly at the scared staff peeping occasionally from their windows, not understanding a word. Whether community treatment orders became law or not, this was an unprecedented show of strength from the grass roots mental health survivor movement, one which went far beyond the more polite, pleading campaigning that had often preceded. It was a 'victory' in itself.

When we'd finished, the media and police went home, the SANE staff remained barricaded in their offices until they were sure the coast was clear, and the rest of us went to the nearest pub. There we celebrated and Pete, Simon, Mark and me resolved to keep up the pressure, intending to launch Mad Pride as soon as possible. Frequent evening meetings continued, part of the frenzied hard work behind the scenes.

The media made much of "*psychiatric patients protesting against a charity that claims it's trying to help them*", and footage of the protest was shown on the news on primetime TV. SANE have never been quite the same since.

Working almost around the clock, splitting up with Mina for a second time, and with my alcohol intake re-escalating I was exhausting myself, and something had to give: namely, my pancreas. I wouldn't recommend acute pancreatitis as a leisure option: it hurts. It appears to be caused usually by severe alcohol misuse, and involves digestive enzymes travelling around the body in the wrong direction and literally digesting parts of the pancreas. It's very often fatal, and women I've met who have both had pancreatitis and given birth have told me that the former is the more painful. For a couple of days in an orthopaedic ward in Homerton Hospital, I genuinely believed I was going to die, but in fact I recovered remarkably quickly. Hospital, though, was a nightmare. They stuck a catheter up my urethra, apparently to make it easier for them to measure the volume of urine I was passing, and I could feel physical pain from it despite the morphine I was being injected with to lessen the pain from my pancreas. I was also attached to an array of other tubes and wires, most of which were connected to a seven-feet tall metal tripod on wheels, which I had to cart along with me whenever I struggled to the stairwell for a fag. I'd never believed it possible to feel so ill and yet still stay alive, and I ran out of tobacco.

The tubes were all that separated the tripod from my veins, but I needed to get to the nearest off licence four hundred yards from the hospital gates. I'd suddenly gone off alcohol, but I was dying for a fag. Breaking the rules, I dragged the tripod with me past the security guards on the gates without them noticing. I'd been on nil by mouth for three days, I was wearing a blood-splattered hospital gown over some of my other clothes and I was finding it a terrible struggle to simply move along, feeling weak and faint. The off licence proprietor looked a little startled when I went inside to get my tobacco surrounded by my mobile fluids in transparent plastic. I can't think why he was so surprised: I discovered later that Homerton Hospital patients quite frequently managed to get to the shop in similar conditions. With difficulty I made my way back to the ward, sorted for snout.

After five days I was disconnected from the machine, still in pain but extremely bored. I'd been dictating instructions to the Southwark Mind staff via my mobile phone, and I was anxious to get back to this work and to the Mad Pride project, both of which I thought were approaching exciting and critical phases. Against medical advice I discharged myself, and had to sign a form forgiving the hospital for any disasters which might result from my premature departure. Reckless and not thinking rationally, I was back at work the next day. I had the first ever Mad Pride event to stage-manage a few days later.

The show took place at the Foundry, a bar in Old Street owned by Bill Drummond of the KLF. It was a suitably dilapidated place, frequented mostly by young artists and musicians including the Libertines and their crew. Foam-protruding sofas lined the walls and there was a gallery in the basement which featured underground proletarian artists at odds with the fashionable Hoxton

MAD PRIDE and VIVA IGUANA present...

AN AFTERNOON OF FOLK MUSIC, STORYTELLING, POETRY AND PUNK ROCK

LIVE at THE FOUNDRY, 84-86 Great Eastern Street, London EC2a 3JL

SUNDAY 20TH JUNE 1999, 3-8 PM.

with:

THE LONG DECLINE
FRANK BANGAY
SARAH O'DRISCOLL & SAM SIDDOL
TED CURTIS
DAVE RUSSELL

ADMISSION: FREE

This event has been organised to launch MAD PRIDE, an organisation dedicated to promoting rights for psychiatric service users and to challenging stereotypes. There will be a bar, and cheap food.

crowd nearby. Rebecca Feiner and her friend Dave ran a weekly Sunday show there, which with their permission Mad Pride gate-crashed for the day. Separately, Rebecca had distinguished herself by putting on her own art exhibition in the Foundry which bravely depicted sexual abuse she'd suffered at the hands of family members as a child. After reading about the show in *Time Out*, her brothers turned up and trashed the exhibits, which Rebecca rebuilt, incorporating some of the damage into the reconstituted pieces so that it acted dialectically with the work.

The headlining band, the Long Decline, was run by Leigh Goorney, whose stage name was Kenny Wisdom. I once ran into him in Borough High Street and became engaged in a conversation about the singer's dental health. His teeth were fucked, and one of the front ones consisted only of a small aluminium stalk protruding from his upper gums, a remnant of a capped tooth which had fallen off. "*Why don't you get your tooth fixed, Leigh?*" I asked him.

"*Because I don't like dentists*" he explained. "*They're all sadistic bastards!*"

"*True, but I've got a capped front tooth myself from falling off a pushbike when I was ten. If it fell out, all the dentist has to do is put a new one back in, it doesn't hurt or nothing.*" I told him this.

"*Yes, but then they might look at my other teeth!*"

He was probably right. Pete, Simon, Mark and me had been talking up the idea of Mad Pride to mental health charities and user groups, envisaging it as a political and artistic weapon which would combine campaigning and demonstrations with high quality performative assertions of radical culture from within the user movement. The SANE demo had been controversial. Many users and workers were uncomfortable with our full-on targeting of a charity, but many more wanted to lend us their weight, sometimes clandestinely. In the past the user movement had sometimes adopted a pleading, "*we're nice people really, please like us*" strategy, whereas we had the idea of saying "*actually, we're complete bastards and we don't care whether you like us or not, we're going to force you to meet our demands anyway*". We had no disrespect for people with sedate outlooks and tastes, not unless they were annoying us, but we felt there was a gap in the market for something more ostentatiously rebellious. It was appropriate, therefore, that the early Mad Pride shows should feature acts principally from out of the punk rock movement.

We'd sent publicity to all of the user groups we'd heard of, and remarkably, some people travelled from as far as Wales to get to the Foundry. It was Sunday 20th June 1999, and the show ran from three until eight in the afternoon. Veteran folk-rock singer-guitarist Dave Russell opened the show, gaining the status of being Mad Pride's first ever live musician. He has a unique and uncanny guitar technique involving fast, complex arpeggios, strange time signatures and wild slide routines which he performs with thimbles over his fingers and his guitar perched horizontally across his lap. Comparable in ability and contemporary to Davy Graham, Dave is one of the great unsung heroes of British pop. Pete Shaughnessy, drunken and hilarious, was master of ceremonies, introducing the show and explaining the previously unheard of concept of Mad Pride; Ted Curtis performed some storytelling; Frank Bangay Tony Palfrey and Dee Light recited poetry; and Sarah O'Driscoll, a torch singer from Leeds with a beautiful, fluty voice sang accompanied by her boyfriend on piano. Headlining act the Long Decline's violinist had left the band shortly before the show, and when Leigh asked me if I knew any other violinists who were at a loose end I suggested Mina, who got the job. Previously the band had featured punk legends Mark Perry and Vic Godard, and in future would boast another two, Jowe Head and Karl Blake, but even without these stars they put on a spiky and accomplished folk-rock performance which went down a storm. I'd only been out of hospital for a few days and it was the first gig I'd ever helped organise without the comfort and reassurance of alcohol. Sobriety felt strange, but the atmosphere at the show led me to believe that it could be start of something important, and in the event I remained sober for a year.

Very shortly prior to this Southwark Mind had held a demo, using Pete's Reclaim Bedlam front, outside the Royal College of Psychiatry in a posh square in central London. We were challenging the continued use of electro-convulsive therapy in the UK, a 'treatment' banned in more civilised nations such as Germany and Norway. ECT, though apparently shocking some people out of depression for a few days, had no long-term benefits and was proven to cause long-term brain damage, with a particular impact on memory. The majority of people given ECT were depressed women over retirement age: we thought it was barbaric and should be banned. After this we held a picnic outside the Imperial War Museum, site of the original Bedlam. Users from

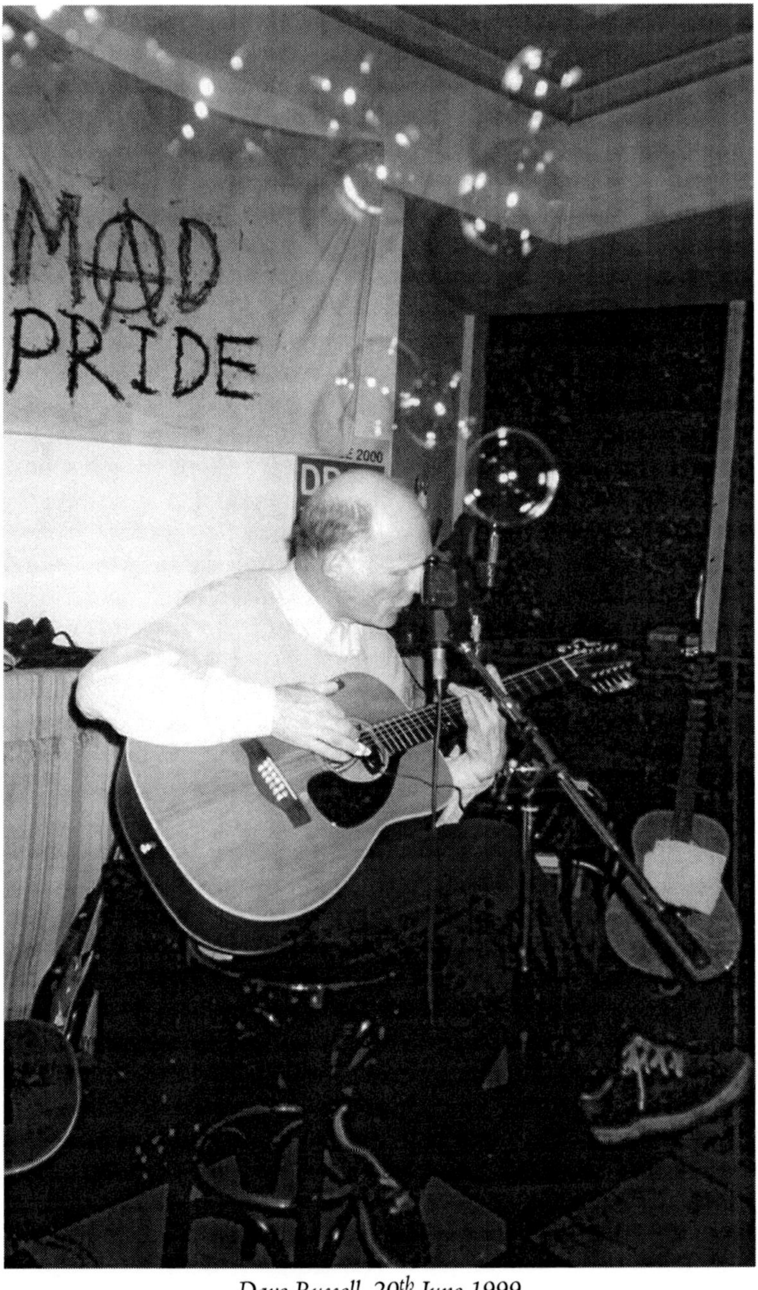

Dave Russell, 20th June 1999

across Britain had turned up to the protest and members of the Welsh contingent, accustomed to institutional and disempowering day centre culture, were outraged that we hadn't provided them with packed lunches for the picnic. We had supplied large quantities of lager, but this wasn't enough for these fruits: they wanted ham sandwiches, wrapped in clingfilm, a Kit-kat and a carton of Ribena. Pete became angry with their learnt dependency and shouted *"what do you think we are, a fucking day centre?"* at them. He strolled off, reappearing minutes later with a bag of fish and chips which he offered to Wales.

"We're not eating that, we want our ham sandwiches!" Wales bleated. Pete drop-kicked the fish and chips towards the Welsh protesters, showering them with salt and vinegar.

Southwark Mind grew at speed, and Mad Pride was urgent, intense and voluntary activity into which I threw myself wholeheartedly, working around the clock for a year as a substitute for overdrinking. Pete Shaughnessy and Simon Barnett took care of the initial media work, Mark Roberts set up a decent website and did the accounts, and to begin with I concentrated on administration, as well as organising concerts to build the profile. The four of us, each with separate, very different skills but with ideals in common which were so compatible that we barely needed to debate them, made a highly effective team. I'd hooked up with Tuba again, who despite being in the SWP was basically stable and sensible, a supportive presence during twelve months of hectic activity.

I'd just co-published Frank Bangay's poetry book, the superb *Naked Songs and Rhythms of Hope*. There was nothing intellectual about Frank's poems, with no attempts at rhymes or cryptic allusions, just the unadulterated heartfelt truth about the nature of the mental health system and everyday struggles to survive. An experienced performer with still-growing popularity, Frank acted on the belief that the best poems had to be immediately accessible when read aloud, their messages clear and direct. And yet there was nothing overly blunt about his material: there was great beauty and wisdom in it, and his rants and vignettes were moving and haunting. I also began planning the anthology *Mad Pride: A Celebration of Mad Culture*, having raised three grand from the Mind Millennium Awards, and after a couple of meetings I recruited Ben Watson, Ted Curtis and Esther Leslie to help me edit it. We contacted friends who we thought could or

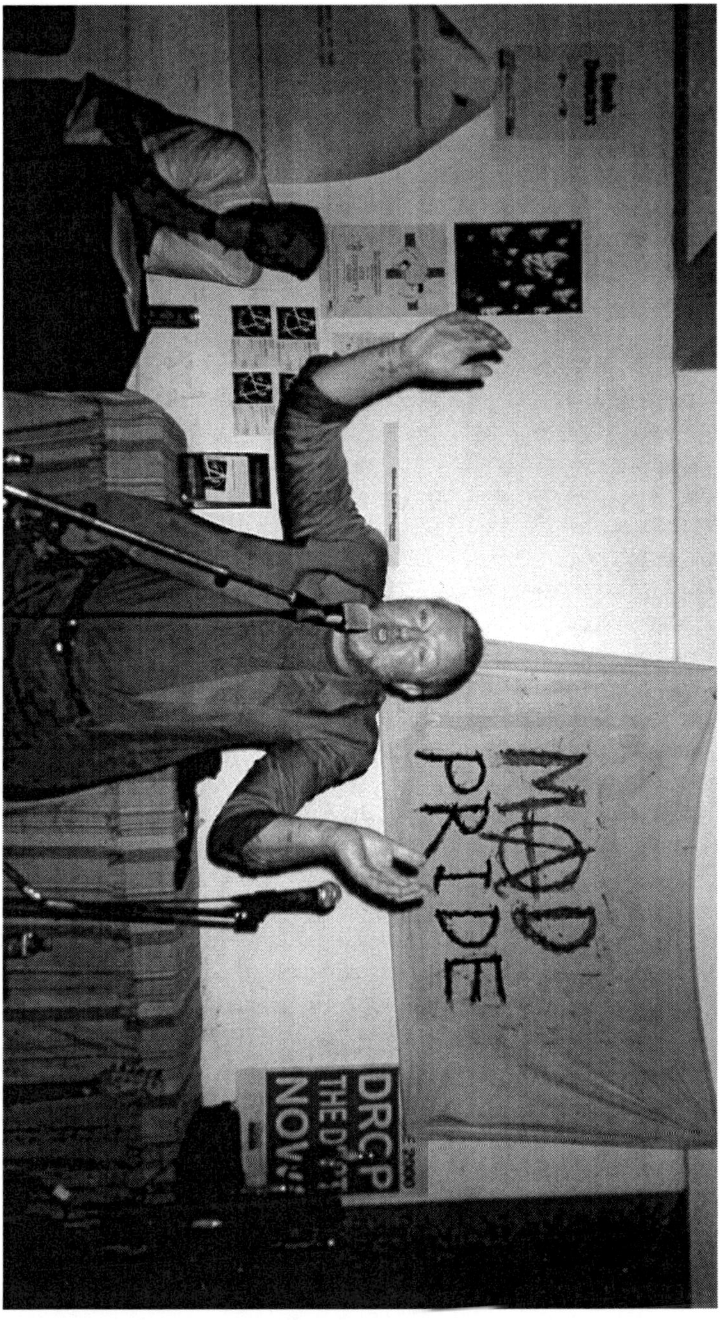

Frank Bangay at the inaugural Mad Pride gig, The Foundry, 20th June 1996

should write, and put the word out further afield that we were looking for material, and as the work flew in it became clear that we were on the verge of curating a rather special book, of far more importance than originally envisaged.

Meanwhile, I organised a conference for Southwark Mind about suicide awareness, which took place upstairs at the Lorrimore in September 1999. Cat Monstersmith had the idea of building a suicide memorial post box, shaped and sized like a regular post box, inviting people to put cards and letters into it for friends and family members of people who had killed themselves. It was a good way for folks to pay respect to their dead and simultaneously 'let go' of some of their grieving, at least in theory. The post box was sealed, making its contents irretrievable, and it had arms reaching from its side, topped with silver plates for people to light candles on. It's a beautiful monument which became peripatetic, spending time in locations such as the Copleston church hall, the Foundry, and one of the atriums at Guy's hospital. Samaritans organisers came to speak at the conference, which looked at the causes of suicide, ways of identifying suicide risks, and methods of preventing suicide. I met Shirley Pearson here for the first time.

The second Mad Pride show was also in September 1999, at the Union Chapel in Highbury, and 300 people attended. Jim MacDougall's band – then called Aural Guerrilla – opened, Jim's vocal improvisations complementing generic punk churned out by musicians he'd met at Core Arts. He'd been given overnight leave from the bin he was in at the time, specially for the show. Then Pauline Bradley, a folk singer-guitarist and Survivors Poetry stalwart who'd previously been in a duo featuring Mina on violin, performed some melodic ballads from an orthodox left-wing perspective, contrasting nicely with Jim's antisocial racket.

Pauline and Mina had once played a full-length set at a party in Stamford Hill put on by members of Socialist Organiser, a bunch of Marxist Labour party entryists. The music had been good, but the event had been notable mostly for the state of the audience. Members of Socialist Organiser, male and female alike, were the ugliest, most physically unattractive group of people in Britain. They made Brighton Labour Briefing look like supermodels. It was barely believable. It was as if Lenin himself had trawled the fringes of the various British socialist caucuses, personally picked the most unfortunate, facially and sartorially

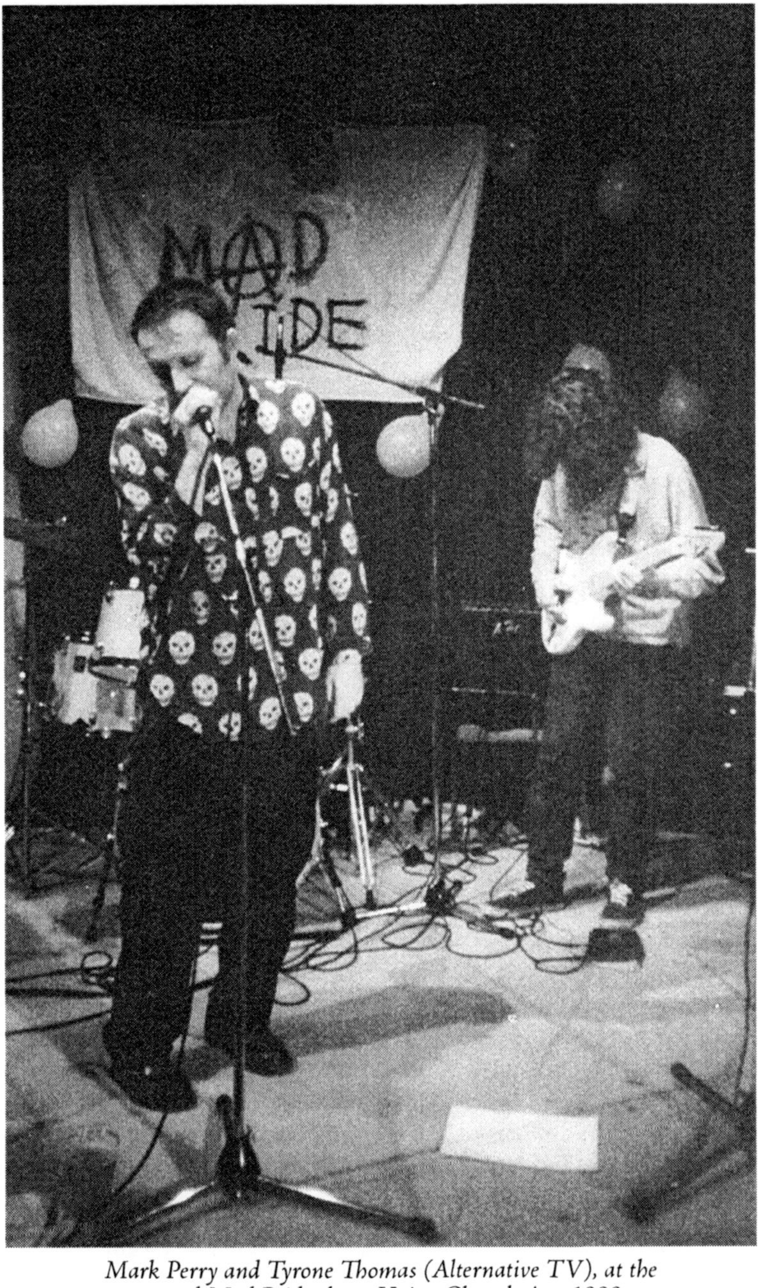

Mark Perry and Tyrone Thomas (Alternative TV), at the second Mad Pride show, Union Chapel, Aug 1999

challenged people in each of these subgroups, and put them all together out of harm's way where they could be invisible to the rest of the movement and to the wider population. Lenin knew that, if it became widely known that the revolution was being planned by such measly, chinless, shapeless, bearded (regardless of gender) specimens of debased humanity with posh voices, the glorious day would never arrive. It made capitalism seem glamorous. It was safer if they could all be kept in one place to interbreed and argue with each other about who was the most politically correct without anyone else having to see them. They were hideous, and after each song they made earnest criticisms of Pauline's lyrics on minor sectarian grounds. Pauline always took things far too seriously, and made the mistake of engaging with these gargoyles, apologetically responding to their whinges and allowing the show to be interrupted by debate. She should have just told them to fuck off. My boss back in those days, Roger Harris, was a member. He obviously hadn't subscribed simply to suss out the talent.

Back at the show in Highbury, Frank Bangay was next, and as always he met with an appreciative reception from the audience of mental health service users and punks, labels which were becoming increasingly interchangeable under the Mad Pride umbrella. He was followed by Ceramic Hobs, an avant-garde punk band from Blackpool based around mad intellectual singer Simon Morris and former Membranes guitarist Stan Batcow, and they had recently released the album *Psychiatric Underground*. Ceramic Hobs had been around in various guises for years without many people noticing, but their ostentatious, theatrical weirdness and gleeful gestures of rebellion earned them immediate star status within the incipient Mad Pride movement.

Finally, Alternative TV headlined. I'd been a fan of theirs from the age of thirteen, and although I'd organised shows for them on previous occasions it was the first time they were specifically booked to play in front of a gang of nutcases. Their leader, Mark Perry, was instinctively cut out for the task, with his lyrics obsessively articulating outsider themes and his performance – as Ben Watson put it in *the Wire* magazine – always demonstrating *"uncanny sensitivity to audience specific situations"*. Mark had never been binned up but clearly knew the score, and ATV's set combined 1970s hits like 'Action Time Vision' and 'Love Lies Limp' with less feted but equally exciting and intelligent songs from their new album *Apollo*. Most memorably, he had his band improvising whilst Frank and Jim did cameo vocal slots, ranting manically into the microphone. Their set finished as usual with the classic angst-punk anthem 'Splitting in Two'. Pete Shaughnessy, blind drunk, was master of ceremonies.

The next Mad Pride show was in October, with anarcho-punk band Citizen Fish headlining at the Garage in Highbury. Although it was nice of them to perform for us and a near sell-out crowd meant that we made some money for a change, their large lumpen punk following overwhelmed the atmosphere, making it simply a Citizen Fish show rather than something bearing any distinctive Mad Pride signature. The Astronauts, the Fish Brothers, Tony Palfrey and Survivors Poetry veteran John Arthur supported.

Events came thick and fast: country-rock legends the Arlenes, led by Core Arts music co-ordinator Big Steve, did a show for us at the Lorrimore day centre in Southwark shortly before Christmas. Big Steve, before he grew to six feet eight inches, had been raised in the rectory next door to the church centre in which the Lorrimore was based, his father having been the vicar. Unfortunately Steve's dad had been caught out by the Sunday scandal-sheet *News of the World* for having an affair with a younger woman behind Steve's mum's back. These days, this wouldn't make the news as papers are concerned only with celebrity misdemeanours, and it is assumed in any case that all vicars give rise to neighbours' daughters being locked up in their vicinity. But in the early seventies it was a front page story, and Steve's dad and family had to move. We billed the show with the strapline 'the prodigal son returns' and it went well, with Jack Hudson, a former Lorrimore Square resident who'd been playing his country-blues back when Steve was a kid, supporting ably. The show was seen mostly by mad Southwark residents and it helped them through some of the Christmas season, normally a dreaded time for mental health service users as the seasonal pressure to live it up tends to amplify misery.

Southwark Mind was still developing nicely with its newsletter appearing monthly, the User Council creaking into action, and numerous local service users signing up to get involved. Mad Pride was even less orthodox and therefore more exciting, though for a time the work overlapped. Debbie McNamara, who had accumulated a lot of experience with Hackney Patients Council as well as through organising shows and fundraising for Survivors Poetry, began to throw herself wholeheartedly into Mad Pride activities, particularly the planning of an open air free festival.

The year 2000 saw the best of Mad Pride's agitation. Lobbies, demonstrations, television appearances and myriad curious magazine and newspaper articles helped spread the concept, with Pete Shaughnessy behind many of the brightest ideas. Some of them were never put into practice: for example, the notion of organising a 'medication strike' to protest against the proposed community treatment orders. This would have involved all mental health service users in Britain stopping taking their antipsychotic drugs at the same time, to create an unprecedented overwhelm of hospital wards and other services. But one idea that did come off was a vigil at Suicide Bridge in Archway which took place late one Saturday night in June in front of TV cameras. At this point, so much was happening so quickly and in such a short space of time that it was difficult to digest it all; indeed, I can't even remember all of it accurately. Pete had the idea for this event after discovering that a local residents' group was organising an 'Archway celebration', casting the bridge as a key neighbourhood attraction. Pete knew that a bridge which had been the scene of so much tragedy, literally dozens of deaths over a period of decades, was nothing to celebrate, and we wanted it demolished. Cat's post box was driven to the vigil and displayed, and Pete and Simon spoke to news reporters about the shockingly high incidence of suicide, and how this was traditionally downplayed in the media in favour of rare high profile cases of psychiatric patients being violent. At one point a small group of local middle-class do-gooders approached us, happy that we were 'joining in' with the Archway celebration. We corrected their false assumption and told them where they could go. Julie Hathaway and Eddie Murray got out their guitars and sang a few tunes at the bus stop on the bridge, and the event was somehow affirmative and heartbreaking at the same time. It was difficult for me to stop thinking all evening about Jo Crane, who had taken her own life from that exact location. Negotiations took place with the Samaritans about setting up a permanent stall there, as they have at Beachy Head, and although this came to nothing, the local council did eventually manage to heighten the railings making it prohibitively difficult for anyone without mountaineering equipment to climb over and chuck themselves onto the tarmac below, where they would be at the mercy of lorries being driven at seventy miles an hour. This happening, attended by around a hundred users, tied together some complex and extreme feelings encompassing sadness, anger, and the desire to assert mad people's strength.

The book *Mad Pride: A Celebration of Mad Culture* came back from the printers in April 2000 and was officially released a little later in a blaze of publicity. It attracted 'book of the week' features in the *Guardian* and the *Big Issue*; a front page leader in the anarchist fortnightly *Freedom*, and a two-page Mad Pride spread in *Time Out* which included a fetching photograph of Simon, Ben, Esther, Debbie and myself standing next to Suicide Bridge. I suspect that the *Time Out* piece may have prompted further suspicion within the mental health voluntary sector that I was some kind of a loose cannon, with some of my statements, including the claim that SANE were 'wankers', perceived by some to be controversial.

Two launch events took place and they were both a laugh. The first was at Compendium, which from the sixties until its sad closure in 2001 was the best book shop in London: fiercely radical and independent, it stocked all sorts of underground literature unavailable anywhere else and promoted every book I was involved with in its window display, selling dozens of each. Mike Hart, one of the shop's managers, had a particular passion for obscure poetry and also loved jazz; he facilitated the launch party, pleased that it was likely to be unorthodox, in keeping with Compendium's reputation as Britain's most cutting edge literary venue, which had played host to star writers including Alexander Trocchi, Samuel Beckett, Stewart Home, William Burroughs and thousands of others.

Some years previously I'd been to the launch do for Mark Perry's book *And God Created Punk*, published by Virgin, and it was a corporate affair in the basement of Helter Skelter music bookshop in Denmark Street, the so-called 'Tin Pan Alley'. At this, scantily clad, pretty young girls wandered around the audience holding large silver platters aloft, head-high with postures that must have been uncomfortable to maintain, on which sat triangle-shaped sandwiches with the crusts cut off and various other posh treats. Given the state of the audience, which included drunken has-beens like Jimmy Pursey and Pete Shelley stealing books and artworks, this was incongruous. Mad Pride's book launch was more in keeping with its crowd, and eschewed the expensive red wine in favour of Tennents Super and Diamond White. Ben Watson and myself had visited a local off licence earlier and purchased two hundred of these super-strength cans. But we did not wish to be irresponsible. We were mindful of the fact that alcohol could have an adverse effect if taken in conjunction with certain varieties of psychiatric medication, and we were also aware that many people there might not have eaten, so to lower the risk factor we also bought a few dozen bags of super-saver crisps from a supermarket.

I thought we'd put together a classic book, certainly the best publication I'd been involved with, and it featured 24 mentally distressed writers, as well as animations by Cat Monstersmith which came to life when readers stared at the pages' corners as they flicked through the book. Those giving readings at this launch, all having written chapters, were Debbie McNamara who was accompanied by a violinist, Chris P. from Camden grunge stars Silverfish helped along by a portable beat box, Terry Conway, Tim Telsa who had miraculously managed to get overnight leave from the Kneesworth hospital specifically to attend, and regular Turkish *Big Issue* contributor Fatma Durmush. After the literature, Julie Hathaway, who had designed and desktop-published the book, got up with her acoustic guitar and performed some of her own folk compositions, finishing with a cover of John Lennon's 'Imagine'. Ben Watson was master of ceremonies, commenting later that, with his impeccable BBC accent, he'd felt a little embarrassed introducing these acts, most of whom had strong, working-class regional accents.

Afterwards we went to the pub and there was a fight. The bitter altercation which took place in the beer garden between punk singer Jim MacDougall and Irish folk singer Eddie Murray was a thoroughly appropriate way to continue the evening's entertainment. They had each drank their way through more than their fair share of Diamond White and Tennents Super, and this combined perfectly with the psychiatric medication and neglect of food to make them argumentative and violent. When Eddie asked Jim for a light for his roll-up, trouble was the only possible outcome.

Jim got his lighter and passed it to Eddie, who lit his fag and pocketed the lighter. A minute later, Jim's own fag ran out and he rolled another, before searching his pockets for the lighter which was no longer there. This search took some time, during which Eddie's fag ran out, leaving the Irishman with no choice but to roll a replacement. Eddie produced a lighter from his pocket, which in fact was a different colour to Jim's lighter, which meant that Eddie was now in possession of two lighters, having had his own all along. After the folk singer lit his fag, Jim asked him for a light. Eddie passed him the lighter; Jim lit the fag and pocketed it. Similar exchanges took place over the next twenty minutes, with the pair repeatedly exchanging lighters and becoming increasingly agitated by being hassled by each other. Eventually a third party, Ben Watson, became involved. Ben did not usually smoke, but having drank several cans of Tennents Super he had decided to let his hair down, and asked Eddie not only for a lighter but also a roll-up, which the Irishman graciously granted him. Ben lit the fag and pocketed the lighter, leaving Eddie and Jim with only one lighter between them. When Eddie next asked Jim for a light, the punk, tired of being pestered, refused on the grounds that he no longer had one. Eddie spent the next few minutes searching his pockets frantically and fruitlessly for his lighter, during which time Jim rolled his next cigarette, and reached for his lighter, which in fact was the original lighter that Eddie had owned. Eddie confronted Jim verbally, accusing him of stealing the lighter, to which Jim responded that he had been in possession of the object all along, and that furthermore, Eddie was a fat Irish cunt who couldn't sing a folk tune to save his life. Eddie objected to this claim, pointing out that Jim was a demented English spastic who had probably never met his father. Jim challenged Eddie to repeat this claim outside, seemingly unaware that the beer garden we were sitting in was outside anyway. Eddie slurred something incomprehensibe under his breath, which Jim took to be a further aspersion on his character. A pint had been bought for Jim when we'd arrived at the pub, but this had ran out, meaning that it had to be topped up with lager left over from the book launch: Jim threw the Tennents Super over Eddie, not only making him wet, but also extinguishing his roll-up. Eddie stood up and shouted something which was unintelligible, but plainly intended as abusive, testing Jim's patience further. The punk grabbed the still-seated Eddie by the lapels and head-butted him, prompting the folkie to fall over backwards and hit his head on the table behind him. As Eddie attempted to bring himself to his feet, Jim followed through with an attempted kick to Eddie's

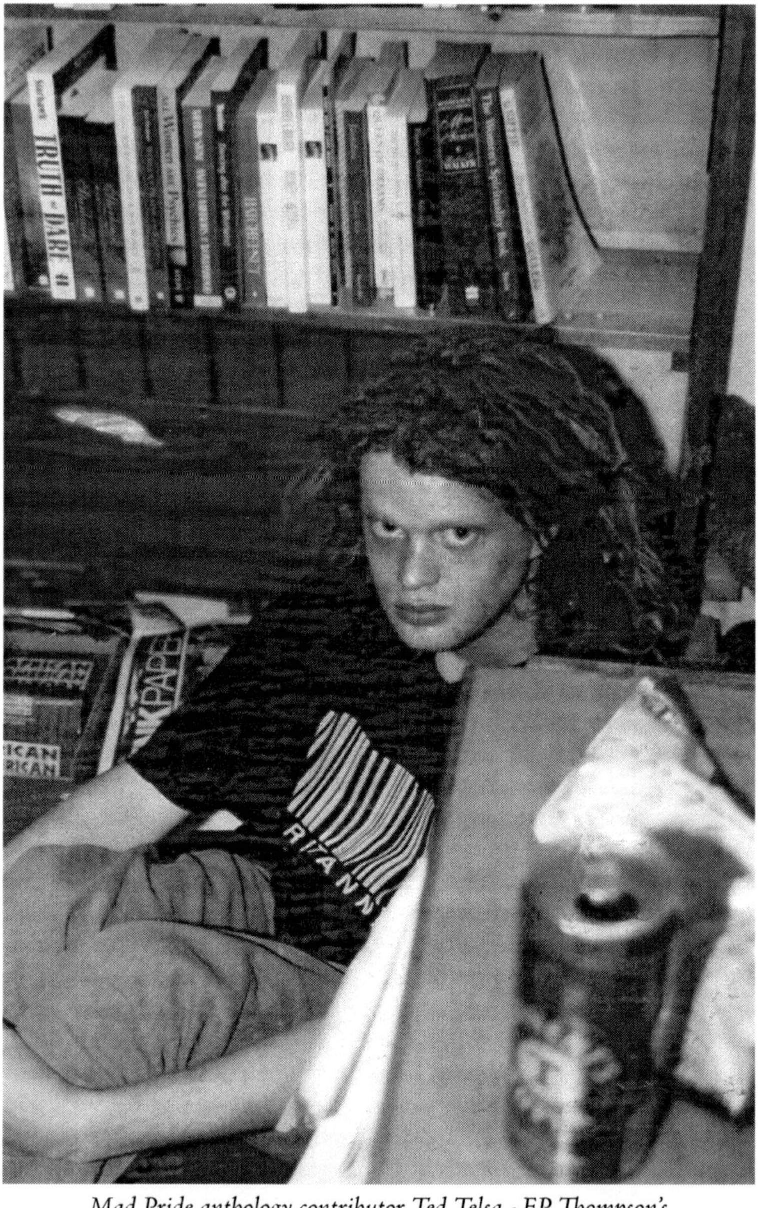

Mad Pride anthology contributor Ted Telsa - EP Thompson's grandson - on escorted leave from Kneesworth Hospital at the book's launch at Compendium Books in May 2000. A famous fight between Jim MacDougall and Eddie Murray took place in the pub later.

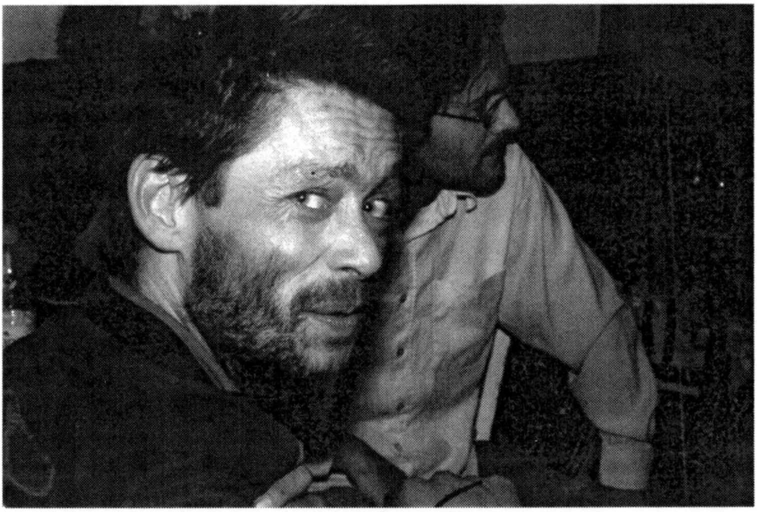

Jim MacDougall

head, which missed, causing Jim to hurt his foot on the nearby thick concrete pot which accommodated a plant. Jim hopped on the spot a few times in pain, and then fell over backwards into a table, knocking over half a dozen pint glasses which spilt half their contents over Eddie who by now, with the aid of the table which he was leaning against to support his weight, was almost upright. Eddie took advantage of Jim's now horizontal position to get in a few kicks of his own, which struck the drunken punk rocker in the ribs, chest and privates, before the Irishman fell over once again into a pile of broken pint glasses. Jim struggled to haul himself to his feet, and then his legs gave way again and he landed on top of Eddie, and the pair had a wrestling match for the next twenty seconds, rolling around in the puddles of beer, fag butts and shards and splinters of shattered glass. One of the bar staff appeared, and some of us thought it wise to separate the wrestlers, haul them to their feet and take them into the street for a while to calm down, in case we were all kicked out. After a few minutes the pair relaxed and we led them back into the beer garden where they sat at a table, chatting amicably, the best of friends. Both of them had already forgotten about the incident, and they had no inkling of where their abundant cuts and bruises had arisen from when they awoke in separate waste skips in Camden's side streets the following morning.

I blamed Ben. If he hadn't taken one of the lighters, then sanity would surely have prevailed. However, by the time the pub closed there were still some cans left from the launch, so we went to the Arlington wet hostel and handed them out to the residents as they stumbled home from the pubs they'd been in. I'd been sober for nearly a year at this stage, and the events of the evening made me feel happy to be one of the responsible people for a change.

The next launch event was back in Chat's Palace, and had more of a rock'n'roll angle. I'd become used to the venue, having not long previously put ATV on there again with some support acts. This show been notable for reactions from feminists, who heckled Jim MacDougall's spoken word pornographic short stories, and applauded dominatrix Deb Percy's equally pornographic stand-up comedy routine. By June 2000, the Mad Pride book's publicity and positive reviews in magazines and newspapers all over Britain was leading to ever-widening public interest in the movement. Contributors Hugh Mulhall and Ted Curtis gave readings, and the now recovered Eddie Murray sang some of his folk songs; it was the first time he'd ever performed amplified. Louise Challice's punk-pop band Hysteria Ward came next. Louise, a veteran from the early eighties Wapping Autonomy Centre, hadn't played live for ten years, having been deterred from performing by the heckling she'd encountered at a show supporting the Stranglers, but the Mad Pride audience was very appreciative and respectful; she looked and sounded like a psychiatric version of Patti Smith. Finally Ceramic Hobs took the stage, delivering an exciting and surprisingly professional set which included Swell Maps, Stooges and Captain Sensible covers as well as their own material; the set was recorded, and later released as a live album entitled *From the Tin City*. Pete and Simon shared the MC duties, drunkenly revelling in the spirit of rebellion and success, and urging the audience to go out and start riots in the name of mental patients' emancipation. *"We're going to fight this fucking system"*, Pete shouted from the stage, pint in one hand, roll-up in the other, *"and we'll fight it all the way, right to the fucking death!"*

He did.

Freak Show

Southwark Mind was still busy but my main passion at this time was for books and pop concerts. The most successful show I've been involved with took place on Saturday July 15th 2000. It was the Mad Pride open air free festival in Clissold Park, Stoke Newington, with bands across two stages and a variety of stalls and tents selling books and food, and there were chill-out spaces, mental health information stalls and a crèche. The advance organisation was hard work: Debbie and myself did most of it, cutting corners wherever possible and breaking every rule in the book. We didn't even bother getting an entertainments licence from the council, which would have been prohibitively expensive. As far as Hackney council was concerned, we were putting together a quiet little picnic for a few regulars from a local day centre. It wasn't until the afternoon before the festival – Bastille Day in fact – that the bureaucrats finally became aware of the advance publicity, which had included an abundance of posters, press coverage and radio reports. And stickers: taking a leaf from Class War's book, we'd printed thousands. They were cheap, they got the word around, it gave expression to our childlike naughtiness to stick them up at bus stops and zebra crossings, and they bore slogans such as 'No government, no mental health problems'. Finally, the council phoned Simon Barnett at five o'clock on the Friday, asking *"what's going on here, then?"* Fortunately for us not much work gets done by Hackney council during evenings and weekends, and pulling the plugs on the show at this late hour would have involved more effort than they were prepared for.

Nikki Sudden and his band the Last Bandits turned up the night before the festival from Berlin where they lived, playing live at Borders book shop in Oxford Street to promote Nikki's new greatest hits album. I'd fallen off the wagon a few days previously using a recent split with Tuba as an excuse, but somehow I managed to transport the drum kit I'd borrowed from Core Arts to the west end for the show. In all the hectic activity, I lost the ride cymbal on the way home afterwards and had to spend eighty quid to replace it.

I'd been a fan of Nikki's since the late seventies, and a friend since I'd interviewed him for a magazine in 1980. I'd loved his band Swell Maps: a spiky, often avant-garde post-punk act balancing wacky humour with an intensity which was disturbing in a way that was difficult to figure. After this lot split up, Nikki pursued a solo career making classic rock'n'roll sounds influenced by Marc Bolan, Johnny Thunders, Bob Dylan and Keith Richards. He had a unique sense of narrative, camp quirkiness and an ear for a telling phrase. On and off he'd also teamed up with a like-minded singer, guitarist, songwriter and reprobate, Birmingham's Dave Kusworth, recording and touring as the Jacobites, whose finest moment was 1985's *Robespierre's Velvet Basement*. Revered by fellow musicians but mostly ignored by the commercial record-buying public, Nikki has left a legacy which will survive long after his chart-bothering contemporaries have been forgotten. He was charming, witty, obsessive and intelligent, and it was always a pleasure to be in his company. It didn't surprise me when Nikki and his band, the best there was from within their chosen dissolute corner of rock'n'roll, sucked the punters towards their stage like a vacuum cleaner and went down a storm at the Mad Pride festival, which nearly never happened. Pete and his fiancée Penny Mount, Nikki's band and me had been up drinking and nattering for most of the night in my flat after Borders, and when it was time to set things up in Clissold Park in the morning most of us were asleep in armchairs, under tables, and anywhere else a space could be found. Debbie had been assigned the task of dealing at the crack of dawn with Hackney Festival Support Group, who had been booked to supply musical equipment and a marquee. She didn't arrive, and if Pete hadn't woken up early after only two hours' sleep and shouted us out of our slumbers, to be on the safe side in case Debbie didn't turn up, the festival would have been cancelled. Pete and I showed up just in time to prevent the Support Group, who had given up on us, from leaving, and they were very annoyed about having had to wait around for the past hour. After we gave them a bribe they begrudgingly set up the stages, finishing the job just in time before the bands and the first punters turned up.

Independent jugglers, ambulant theatre groups, fire-eaters and falafel salespeople jostled for space between stalls, tents and impromptu samba chains. I was more interested in the bands. The largest stage, which was a design feature of the park and even had its own power supply, was stage-managed by Pete, who was also master of ceremonies there. By the time the second act had started he was, I'm told, already drunk, and he was launching into heartfelt tirades defending mental health service users with sophisticated arguments such as *"sane people can fuck off!"* By the time park attendants appeared and advised him to watch his language, over a thousand people were gazing towards the stage enjoying the music and waiting to be verbally abused by Pete. There was a children's play area nearby and anxious parents were casting funny looks in Pete's direction, a little intimidated and keeping their kids safely on their leads. The old bill were milling around too, cautiously, trying not to exacerbate tensions, but ready to pounce at a moment's notice. The first band on this stage were Pink, who were rock'n'rolling sixteen-year old girls with guitars who we'd allowed to play only because they'd lent us some of their back line. Leviant were another feature of the afternoon's entertainment, a truly dreadful heavy metal band who we'd grudgingly put on the bill only to shut Debbie up, as for some reason she'd spent months insisting aggressively and at every opportunity that they should play. Neither of these bands were up to the usual Mad Pride standards, and Leviant actually prompted a mass exodus from the park, their infantile headbanging being so excruciatingly atrocious. Fortunately the deserters either returned or were replaced by new people, and sharp sets from the Fish Brothers, Gertrude, the Stratford Mercenaries and PAIN more than made up for the earlier disappointments.

Simon was master of ceremonies at the second stage, which had been assembled for the day beneath a temporary marquee, and I stage-managed the proceedings. As well as Nikki and his band, there were performances by the Astronauts, Hysteria Ward, Ceramic Hobs, the Long Decline, poets Julie McNamara and Frank Bangay, and most memorably of all, Alabama 3.

Alabama 3 were a self-styled 'country techno' act from Brixton whose records were overproduced, but they had a reputation as a hot live proposition. They'd had two hit singles, 'Woke up One Morning' which had earned them a lot of royalties as theme tune for telly programme the *Sopranos*, and another song entitled 'Ain't Going to Goa'. At the time it felt like a coup to secure their services, but dealing with proper pop stars was an eye-opening experience. Their record company and publishers were mindful of the fact that a new album was due for release, and that involvement with a group of mental patients called Mad Pride could, at the time, backfire commercially, especially given the whispers surrounding the band. Alabama 3 were reluctant to openly disobey their handlers' wishes because they owed them over a million quid which the band had squandered on drugs, hospital and rehab bills, publicity campaigns, dog tracks and extensive studio time. They wanted to play anyway, but only if they were billed as Larry Love's Showband. Word slipped out and sections of the media trailed Alabama 3's appearance, leading to them being told off by their bosses. Torn between conflicting demands and seemingly confused, they repeatedly told us that they were pulling out of the festival, only to phone us minutes later changing their minds, and we weren't certain they'd play until they actually turned up on the day. Rob Spragg, their lead singer, was a clever and basically decent guy, but success and too much cocaine, an inauspicious combination, had gone to his head a little and unlike most musicians I'd worked with, he came across as something of a prima donna. He was very specific about his rider. It had to be a crate of Stella, two bottles of vodka, cheese sandwiches and several grams of cocaine. Rob dabbed at the powder without offering any to me, and ranted and waved his arms around theatrically and at length outside the transit van containing the bands' riders, parked conveniently next to the marquee. The show had really fucked him up, he kept repeating, over and over and over again. His relationship with his record company, the bookings agency, his publishing company: all of it was ruined, he imagined, all because of us. In fact, it transpired that his sister had attempted suicide a couple of days before the

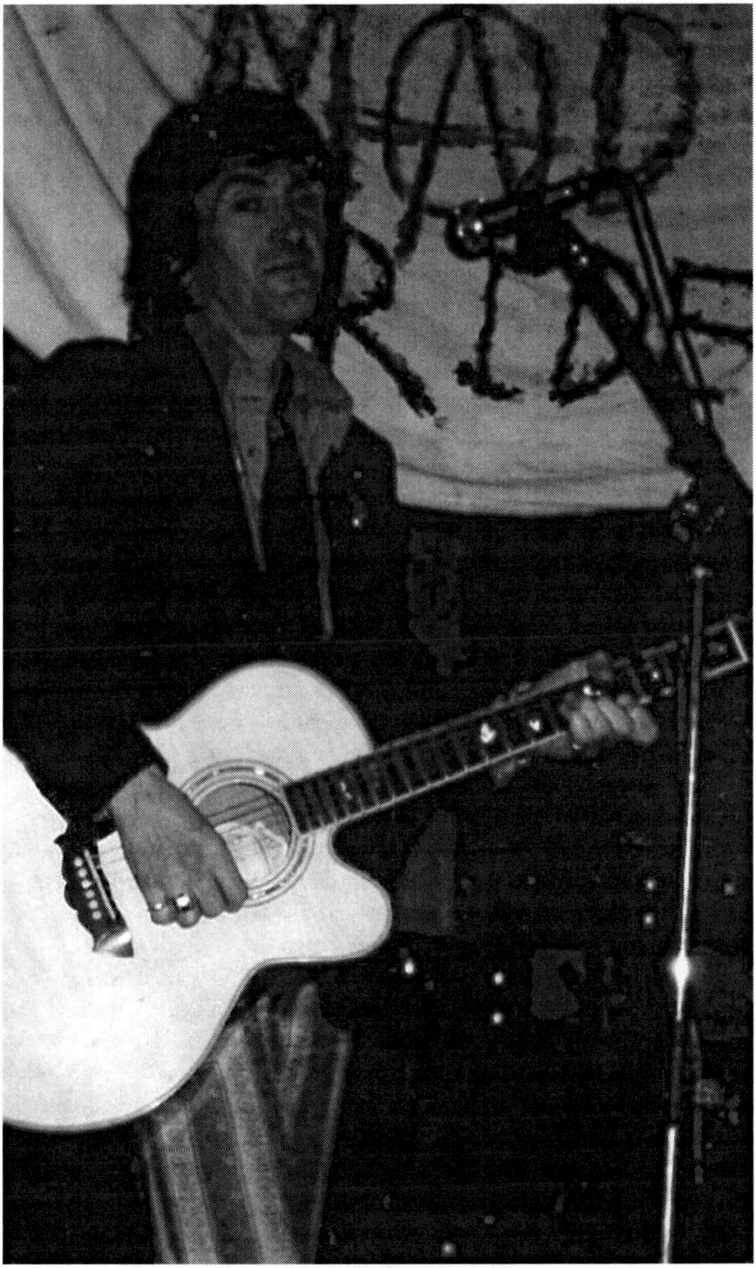

Nikki Sudden, Mad Pride

festival, and this had understandably caused him a great deal of distress. In the event he put on a fantastic show.

The stage was running late and a couple of songs into Alabama 3's set, the Hackney Festival Support Group arrived, hassling us and wanting their equipment back. They were hoping to dismantle the stage and marquee as quickly as possible so that they could get home in time for *Match of the Day*.

An argument followed between the support group's front man and a drunken, belligerent Pete Shaughnessy, who felt affronted by what he saw as the guy's heavy-handed manner. The row culminated in Pete calling the bloke a cunt and punching him in the face, and the bastard went down spitting out blood and broken teeth. The Support Group retaliated by turning off the generator, instantly killing off Alabama 3's amplification. Undeterred, the band continued acoustically, drawing the audience closer to them in a tight mass so that they could hear. *"Can you take this tent down a bit more quietly please? We're doing a show here"*, Rob suggested diplomatically as the tent and then the stage were dismantled around them and the music played on. Once the gear had been taken away the band, like pied pipers, led the few hundred remaining fans towards the park's perimeter fence, against which the musicians leant and carried on performing for an hour or so, finishing their set with the timeless country classic 'The Old Purple Tin'.

The entire event set us back three grand, around a tenth of what a festival of such a size would normally cost to stage. Ignoring statutory health and safety regulations, not being insured, avoiding council and police costs, and paying the bands nothing except for their travelling expenses and a few cans of lager meant that the day was as cheap as it was cheerful.

After we packed up and watched the old bill hassle a remaining drinking school lighting a bonfire in the park's sandpit, the organisers went to one of Stoke Newington Church Street's notorious Indian restaurants for dinner, paid for out of the collection bucket. As we walked we bumped into the lead singer of the Stratford Mercenaries. We'd expected former Crass singer Steve Ignorant to sing for this band, but as it turned out he'd resigned a few weeks previously and been replaced by a younger man, whose girlfriend was American. Pete Shaughnessy didn't like Americans. *"You're a cunt!"* Pete told the singer as he grabbed him by the collar. *"You're a fucking American lover!"*

"Excuse me", the bemused punk vocalist replied, *"we've just done a show for you lot without being paid a penny, and now you're calling me a cunt!"*

"That's because you're a cunt!" Pete explained, squaring up further. The rest of us separated the pair before Pete could do any damage: he was twice the trembling Stratford Mercenary's size. Pete's mood hadn't changed much by the time we reached the restaurant. For no clear reason, Pete insisted on repeatedly calling the waiter a cunt and threatening to deck the guy. The rest of us used our diplomatic skills, remarkably managing to finish our meals and pay the bill before being ejected without an actual fight breaking out. Pete, who was upset that we hadn't taken his side in the restaurant and helped to kick shit out of the cunt, stormed off sulking, eventually reappearing at my flat at six in the morning, slightly more sober. His behaviour, out of character, was an early indication of how stressful it had actually been to organise and manage the festival, and the related Mad Pride activities taking place concurrently. Caught in the thick of it, we hadn't taken stock of the toll the work was taking on us. Simon Barnett, Mark Roberts and, though she would dislike seeing it described us such, Debbie McNamara lapsed into their own unique varieties of psychosis after the festival, while I retreated further into alcohol abuse and depression. This happened very quickly, and life would never quite be the same for any of us again.

Unwisely, exhausted as we were, we agreed to become involved with another festival, Hackney Volcano, a few weeks later on Hackney Marshes. Debbie had already been meeting with some of the organisers, and I'd been approached separately by a chick looking for Mad Pride performers for her music and poetry tent. I contacted some of my musician friends asking them to play this tent, expecting this to be straightforward, but Debbie – manic without realising it at the time or afterwards – had other ideas, and she began phoning musicians in the middle of the night, transferring them from one tent bill and time slot to another, without informing either me or those managing the different tents.

Where various performers should be and at which times, running orders, and requirements for amplifiers, microphones and other musical equipment became increasingly confused. I became aware of this when several musicians, and the tent organiser who'd originally approached me, telephoned me exasperated, complaining about feeling bullied by Debbie and appearing to regret ever having heard of Mad Pride. I shared my concern with some of them that Debbie wasn't herself, and tried to rescue some of the planning which had fallen into chaos. This led to Debbie becoming verbally aggressive towards me. Not feeling too well myself, not wishing to further antagonise her and not strictly needing the anxiety being provoked, I decided to stand back and let her get on with it. Predictably, Mad Pride's parts of the festival were shambolic. Leviant, quite possibly the worst rock band of all time, the truly awful heavy metal trio whose only fan was Debbie, had somehow wound up on the largest of the stages, and managed to send several hundred spectators fleeing to the opposite end of Hackney Marshes despite having to truncate their set due to their having turned up half an hour after they'd been due to start. The stage run by the woman who'd contacted me didn't even have a microphone stand, making it especially difficult for musicians who expected to sing and play guitar at the same time. The Long Decline, Dave Russell, Louise Challice, the Fish Brothers and the Astronauts gamely did their best, not really sure where they were supposed to be playing but settling on this tent because they recognised a few people hanging around; but the sound equipment was woefully inadequate and the afternoon was an embarrassment for us. Pete even had to sit in front of Louise, partly obscuring her from the sparse audience during her entire set so that he could hold the microphone towards her mouth as she sang, her hands being occupied with her guitar. Mad Pride made numerous sheepish apologies afterwards. In her grandiose confusion, Debbie considered this debacle to be a complete success.

A few days later, a debriefing meeting was held at Pumpkins for the Clissold Park festival organisers and numerous volunteers who had helped. It seemed that most of us were losing the plot, and the exercise wasn't very constructive. Debbie challenged me rather aggressively for suggesting she was unwell. I lost my temper, which is rare for me, and stormed out pursued by Pete, who tried to calm me. Mad Pride was starting to unravel. Yet another book launch event took place at Wood Green library in September, with Terry, Ben, Ted and myself delivering readings and hosting a discussion, but my heart wasn't in it. Esther filmed the event, and it was embarrassing to see the video later:

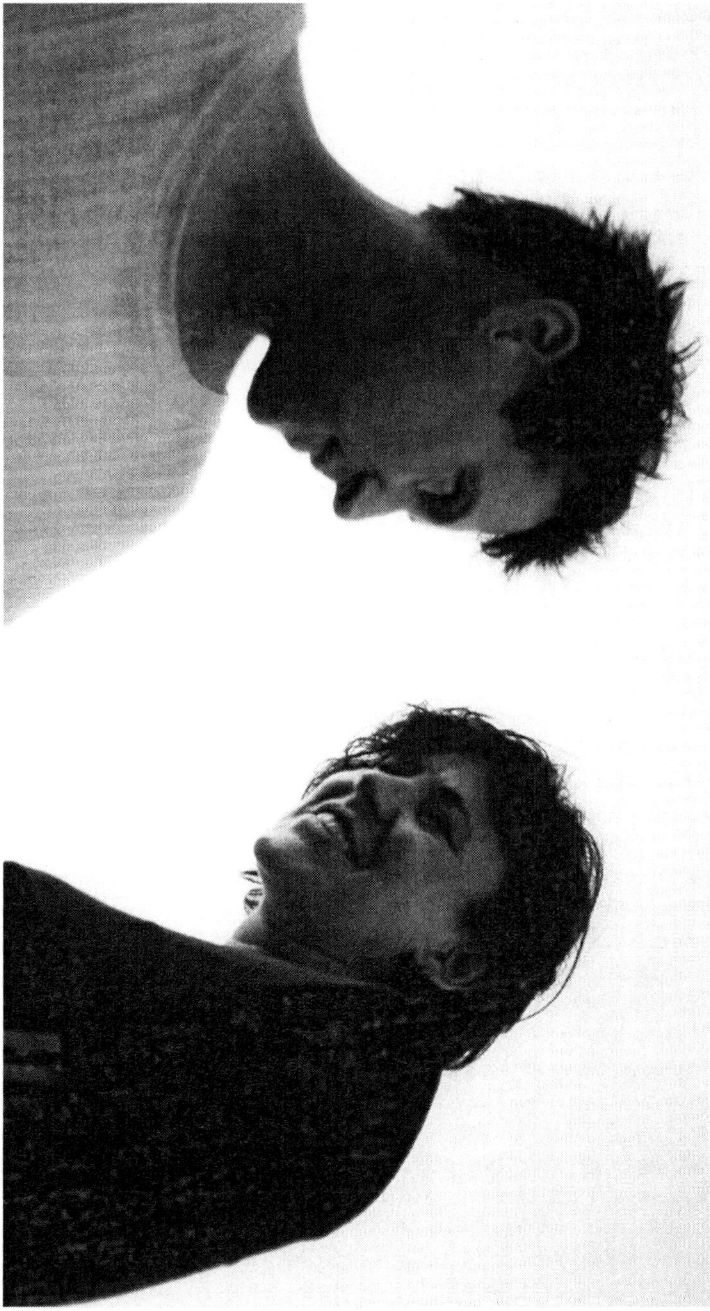

Rob Dellar and Gini Simpson

I looked tired and puffy-faced, and I was visibly trembling with DTs which the can concealed beneath the bench on stage wasn't alleviating quickly enough.

In December that year, Cat Monstersmith introduced me to Hackney artist Gini Simpson, thinking we'd get on. She was right, and a relationship began which was hard work but never dull. As well as being a performance artist and organiser she worked as an art director for an advertising agency, and had been a child protection social worker in one of her more savoury past lives. Gini was still traumatised following the breakdown of a disastrous affair with a guy named Miles, and although I avoided hard drugs, substance misuse was a permanent feature of the time we spent together. Nevertheless, Gini was ablaze with wild energy, creativity and blinding intelligence, and after five months of feeling as if I was in a virtual stupor, I felt enlivened.

Mad Pride had made its name and offshoots were appearing all over the world, but in its initial configuration it was slowing down. I was exhausted and intoxicated. Simon had relocated for a while to Manchester to live with a chick he'd made pregnant at the most recent Mind Annual Conference behind his long-term partner Corrina's back. Simon hardly knew the baby's mother and eventually returned to Corrina with his tail between his legs. Pete was in the process of moving to Worthing, where he married Penny Mount on December 17th, 2000, in what best man Simon described as *"the world's first* Mad Pride *wedding"*. Mark was psychotic. Debbie had dreams of attracting hundreds of thousands of members of the public to the next open-air festival, which never happened, in Brockwell Park the following summer, which would be headlined by Leviant who would be world-famous by then. We tried to integrate new blood into the group and Jim Edwards took the lead in organising a January show at the squatted Button Factory in Brixton headlined by Head Jam, but this was poorly attended. Simon and Pete kept busy, organising shows up north and in Brighton with some success, helping to further spread the word outside London, and they also spoke through the media and at conferences. Southwark Mind was still going strong and we'd recently employed Jolie Goodman and Teresa Priest as paid workers, strengthening the team invaluably. A second edition of the Mad Pride anthology was published by Ron Coleman's Handsell company, which promptly went into liquidation, leaving half the print run tied up with firms of solicitors deciding which creditors to prioritise.

Me and Simon decided to release a studio compilation album of 'Mad Pride bands'. The first release on the newly established Mad Pride Records imprint was called *Nutters with Attitude*, and its release in September 2001 stimulated a relatively minor resurgence of activity. The album, I thought, contained a good selection of punk, folk and country tunes played by musicians who'd worked with Mad Pride and who were mostly psychiatric service users. As I put it on the sleeve notes, none of the performers were *"exactly the full ticket"*. This comment wound up folk singer Eddie Murray, whose cover of the old Bobby Sands chestnut 'I Wish I Was Back Home in Derry' was included. I explained to Eddie that my flippant use of words and terms traditionally regarded as discriminatory was, in fact, part of an attempt to subvert and reclaim language surrounding mental health issues. I thought that words derived their meanings primarily from the contexts in which they were used, and that each time new politically correct words meaning 'nutter' were introduced, the prejudice would follow, and therefore all of these labels were fair game for humour and verbal experimentation. Eddie wasn't having any of this. *"It's all right for people like you, sitting in your ivory tower"*, he told me, demanding that the entire pressing should be scrapped and reissued with new packaging. He mellowed later, to the extent that he formed a duo with a mandolin player, James, actually called the Full Ticket, who went on to release a fine Irish folk album called *Sound as a Euro*.

As with all compilation albums, different people had vastly contrasting opinions about the material on *Nutters with Attitude*, all preferring different tracks. I had a few favourites: Hysteria Ward's 'Owl Walk' was distressed, exciting and tuneful punk, while 'Mellow My Madness' by DJ Unfit For Work, as Phil Murphy had by now taken to calling himself, was a beautiful electro-ballad, a personal take on mental distress which was heartbreaking but – unlike some of Phil's earlier songs – carried a strong message of survival and hope. It helped that some of the less successful acts on the record contributed their best songs. The album's highlight, however, was 'Make Mine a Large One' by Ceramic Hobs. It was funny, angry and preposterously tasteless.

A few years previously seventeen year old northerner Chris Hartley had been murdered and decapitated in Blackpool, ap-

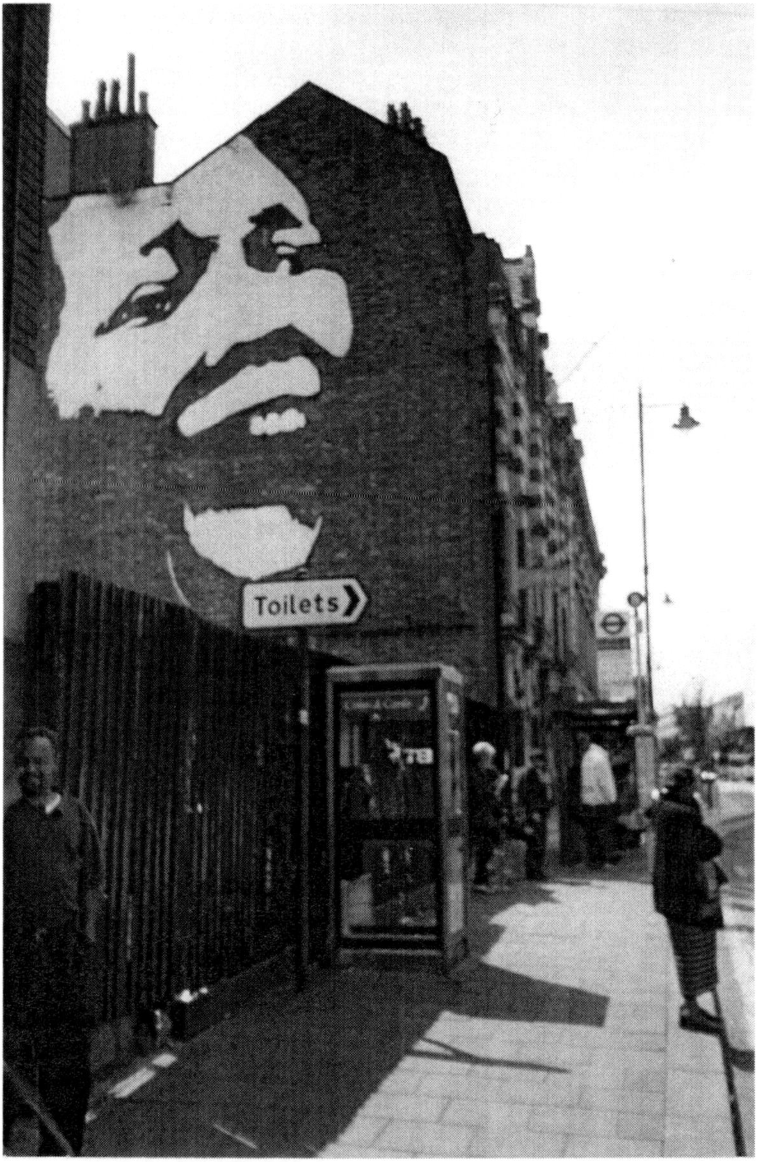

Some Hackney character murdered a tramp and buried the body in a basement in London Fields shortly before painting this mural opposite Hackney Town Hall, which we used for the sleeve of the Mad Pride CD Nutters With Attitude. The character later found religion, confessed and demanded to be executed.

parently by a man named Kevin Diamond who had thrown the severed head into a wheelie bin; Diamond was subsequently labelled with paranoid schizophrenia and carted off to Rampton. But Ceramic Hobs thought they'd discovered the true story behind the disinformation propagated by the media and criminal justice system. *Make Mine a Large One*, narrated by the murderer as role-played by singer Simon Morris, revealed that Diamond had in fact been stitched up to cover for the fact that Hartley had been bumped off by the occult branch of the British intelligence services. Blackpool had been under psychic attack, and it had been necessary for the secret state to offer Hartley's severed head as a sacrifice to dark unknown forces, burying *"the fucking head"*, as Simon repeatedly called it in the song, in a specific ritual location to protect the borough of Blackpool. I'm not sure what Chris Hartley's parents would have made of this track, which I thought would be interpreted as an ironic critique of the media myth that those labelled mad were routinely dangerous, violent and homicidal. *Make Mine a Large One* amplified this stereotype to such an exaggerated extent that it made the stereotype seem ridiculous, taking the piss out of anyone who could believe such nonsense. We knew full well that not everyone would see it that way, and circulated a mischievous press release headlined *"Sick Mad Pride band glorify murder"*, which we hoped would kick off a scandal in the tabloids leading to an increase in record sales.

The promotional video raised the stakes further. Gini, a talented film-maker, and her work colleague James Jacobs, travelled to Blackpool a few times shooting footage and hanging around with the band. The video was nearly as tasteless as the song itself, but our marketing strategy failed to capture popular attention, partly because the contemporaneous September 11th attacks made other distractions less newsworthy by comparison. Even specialist mental health magazines like *Open Mind* for the most part ignored the album, and indeed much of Mad Pride's agitation, finding it too confrontational. A launch occurred at the Garage, Highbury, in October 2001, with a screening of the video and sets from some usual suspects: Alternative TV, Ceramic Hobs, and Skinny Millionaires. The show was good but not spectacular, and the album didn't fare as well as the book, which continued to sell, as did Mad Pride t-shirts. Penny Mount had designed our logo, the name scrawled in scratchy capital letters with the 'a' in 'mad' encircled, as in an anarchy symbol. Anarchism, for us, was more of a fashion statement than a serious expression of intent, but the use of the symbol put mental health issues into a different light by contextualising them within an image normally considered rebellious. When we manufactured t-shirts bearing the logo we sold hundreds in all shapes and sizes, particularly extra-large, since most of our audience had large bellies announcing the ingestion of unfeasible quantities of anti-psychotic medication and lager. The shirt became an indispensable fashion accessory, even amongst people who weren't aware that it referred to a mental health campaign.

Southwark Mind had splashed out on its own PA as it generated its own art and performance events. The first show attributed to 'Southwark Mind Arts Collective' happened in the summer of 2001 in Chumleigh Gardens, a secluded part of Burgess Park in Camberwell which had a delightful selection of tropical plants, a pond and a greasy spoon caff. Country-rocker Alan Tyler played an acoustic set; Sean O'Reilly, Southwark Mind chair at the time, his friend Jenny Yorke and other musicians performed some lively, up-tempo instrumental folk using the moniker Spare Change; and Tony Palfrey was MC, also singing a few of his own camp pop songs. Serious campaigning persisted but I was tiring of it a little, and the playful side of the mental health survivor scene started to feel more meaningful than the serious hard graft.

Love and a Molotov Cocktail

I've always found riots exciting. They can evoke primal, ego-loss situations where, at best, a mob becomes at one and anger erupts into hilarity. I've never liked seeing people being hurt, not even policemen, but property – specifically symbols of capitalism like banks, butchers' shops, building societies, corporate fast food outlets and posh cars – is fair game. I'd participated in more riots over the years than many people had eaten hot dinners, dating back to the Stop the City events in the early 1980s where anarcho-punks and like-minded individuals, pre-Class War, would descend on central London with the sole intention of trashing as many corporate buildings as possible. There's nothing like watching a cascade of shards and splinters of shattered glass exploding from the point of impact when a well-aimed beer bottle strikes an insurance company's head office window. Reclaim the Streets happenings, as well as numerous situations over the years protesting against the Poll Tax, Criminal Justice Bill and various other excuses, were always good for a laugh, but my favourite riots were the spontaneous ones, expressions of joy as much as dissatisfaction, which involved no planning or forethought and which therefore could not be hi-jacked by the SWP and similar organisations. The police, likewise, could not be forewarned.

One of the best was the Arsenal riot of 1998. Me and Tuba had attended an open-air rock festival in Finsbury Park one afternoon, the same day that Arsenal were playing Everton in a home match that, if they won, would confirm them as Premiership champions that year. We left the festival when we became bored of it, and went into an African cafeteria round the corner in Stroud Green Road for dinner. By the time we left the place the junction next to Finsbury Park tube station and the streets around it were swarming with Arsenal, jubilant at their team's triumph. The pubs were overflowing, and the off-licences had been drained of their stock. Arsenal had even hi-jacked a double decker bus and used it to barricade Stroud Green Road so that no traffic could pass, and the cars trapped in the area were showered with lager by hordes of football supporters clearly in a very good mood. A thug, head shaven, tattoos, white t-shirt and blue track suit bottoms with white stripes down the side, approached me and locked me in a bear hug happily. *"Good luck to you, mate!"* he told me. *"Good luck to your bird and all!"* The atmosphere was one of peace and love, and tens of thousands of neighbours emerged from their homes to augment a similar quantity of inebriates who'd streamed out of the Highbury stadium, victorious. Presently, the riot police arrived and before we knew it thousands of football celebrants were kettled into a mile-square area of Islington at the north end of Finsbury Park, side-street exit routes blocked by rows of old bill with shields, helmets and batons who could do nothing to dampen the mood. For hours, Arsenal, trapped, threw empty lager bottles, waste bins, rocks, pint glasses and anything else that came to hand at the cops whilst chanting football slogans. It was as intense as anything Reclaim the Streets ever organised, and had the advantage of occurring totally by surprise. If Everton had won, it might never have happened. Eventually the crowd dispersed, people were allowed to file singly through gaps in the police line in dribs and drabs, and Arsenal and I left the area in a good mood. The riot caused significant damage and disruption, but received no press coverage to speak of, unlike the comparatively minor Mayday riots in years shortly to come which, organised and attended by people with politically radical agendas, were identified by politicians and the media as being more of a serious threat.

Another top spot of bother was the famous Samuel Pepys riot of 2001. Hackney scenester Lucy Teather had organised an open-air free festival in London Fields, celebrating the traditions of the park itself, and among the performers were the Astronauts, country-rockers the John Wayne Army, and a local singing bus-conductor who'd had a number one hit single in South Africa with a cheesy cover version of 'My Boy Lollipop'. At the time, Hackney Council was in the process of 'regenerating' much of the centre of the borough, and this included the refurbishment of the Hackney Empire; the establishment of the ill-fated Ocean venue opposite the town hall; and the summary displacement of pubs and small businesses representative of those actually living in the area. The majority of Hackney's residents were unemployed and living in badly maintained estates combining medium rise blocks and full-on skyscrapers. The tower where Gini lived was typical of local living conditions. The family who lived in the flat directly beneath her held nightly competitions with each other to see which of their sound systems could drown out the others most effectively; typically, three separate rap numbers would be playing at the same time at full volume between midnight and six in the morning. The stairwells and corridors were littered with beer cans, empty chicken and chips cartons, discarded bacon rinds, syringes and used condoms. Owing to endemic local poverty condoms were, like cigarettes, sold to children as 'singles' at the nearby off licence. Kids lurked in the corners shooting heroin instead of going to school. The tower was also blighted by a local 'shit man', who I believed to be a character I remembered from Homerton Friends Lodge and who was living in a ground floor flat. Tom – for this was his name – was clearly unwell, and had developed a habit of saving his excrement until he had amassed a satisfactory amount of the stuff, after which he would smear it liberally over the interiors of the two lifts, and all over the buttons outside used to summon them. This annoyed the residents, particularly those on the upper floors who were disabled or who had prams and heavy bags of shopping, After a while a note was pinned to the door of Tom's flat with a knife, informing him that *"we know who you are"* and that he should expect to be stabbed no fewer than twenty-seven times, a number which may or may not have been significant. I contacted Tom's social worker but, overworked, he was reluctant to intervene, and I've no idea who won the argument between the shit man and local vigilantes after Gini eventually moved out.

This was the reality Hackney Council tried to hide when they closed down the Samuel Pepys. Next door to the Empire, it was a popular and long-standing boozer frequented by those living in the area, an authentic manifestation of local culture. It was affordable, unlike the posh wine bars and arts venues earmarked to replace it and give Hackney a façade of middle-class respectability. By complete co-incidence, the last night of the Pepys prior to its closure took place on the day of Lucy's London Fieldsfest, and inevitably the crowd moved from the park to the pub in the evening after the bands had finished. The pub was heaving, with approximately a thousand pissed-up punters spilling out into the square in front of the Town Hall next door. The night was hot, the crowd was angry about yuppie gentrification, and revolution was in the air. As last orders approached, a spontaneous collective decision was made to break into the town hall as a protest and show of strength. This was duly achieved by using brute force to batter down the front door and dozens of inebriates piled in, kicking their way into bureaucrats' offices and flinging paperwork around wantonly until the riot cops arrived. Gradually the protestors filed out of the town hall and a stand-off ensued until seven o'clock in the morning, with a row of armoured police standing across the steps protecting the municipal building from the rest of us as we jeered and threw empty bottles at the bastards. A celebration at the Hackney Empire was taking place concurrently, with dignitaries and celebrities living it up with champagne and canapés to commemorate its temporary closure for refurbishment beginning the following day. Gini and myself located a side-entrance and found ourselves behind the bar with low-paid, disaffected staff about to be made redundant, and they were happy to give us free crates of bottled lager, which the rioters drank before flinging the empties in the appropriate direction. Remarkably there were few arrests, though I was very fortunate to avoid being one of them. Gini, her flatmate Annabelle and me were required to outrun a gang of helmeted robots after we got lippy with them. Weighed down by riot gear, the cops were less fleet-footed and more flat-footed than would otherwise have been the case. Another local bar, the Old Ship, was hosting a lock-in, and seeing us being pursued, the staff briefly unlocked the back door in Sylvester Passage to allow us in, quickly bolting it behind us to thwart the filth. We relaxed safely and in good company until lunch time, exhilarated by one of the best spontaneous combustions in which we'd had the pleasure to take part.

Around the same time the second anniversary Mad Pride show occurred, in the Foundry where it had all started. Tried and tested usual suspects performed: Nikki Sudden headlining, with slots by the Astronauts, Frank Bangay, Julie Hathaway, Louise Challice and anti-psychiatrist from the sixties Steve Ticktin. It was a good show, but the unravelling of Mad Pride behind the scenes was taking up a fair amount of energy. It had been Mark Roberts' idea to make Mad Pride a company limited by guarantee, primarily to patent the name. Alarm bells had sounded at the time, as I was aware that running a company entailed keeping detailed accounts and filling in fairly complex annual return forms for Companies House and the Inland Revenue. In spite of the fact that Mark and Simon had failed to keep up with the company paperwork for the by then as good as defunct Survivors Speak Out, leading to the group being deregistered and potentially putting its officers at risk, I had initially gone along with the idea to keep Mark happy, surmising that I'd be able to chase up relevant people for paperwork when needed. This proved difficult: my own energy was lessening, Mark's mental health had deteriorated and his ability to function had fallen. The Mad Pride website, which initially he'd set up brilliantly, disappeared when he failed to pay the annual host server's fee, and he refused to share with the rest of us the information we needed to keep the site up and running ourselves, in the belief that he'd pick things up in time and be able to maintain control of it himself. In the event, somebody entirely unknown to us took over our original website address and replaced its original content with hard-core porn images, which didn't make us appear too clever.

Mark eventually got the boot from his job, which prior to this spell of difficulties he'd by all accounts been very good at, running a 'common agendas' project at Greater London Action for Disabilities, a Brixton-based rights, campaigning and support group within which he had been able to highlight the links between mental health issues and wider, generic disability politics. During a protracted withdrawal from his post he took with him and sat on essential information, such as mailing lists, leaving a hole in the materials required for other people to keep the project running. Such was also the case with regards to Mad Pride's accounts and related paperwork, which Mark had agreed to lead. We were aware of the distinct possibility of legal action and huge fines if we failed to return the material required by law from limited companies. Simon, although he too was losing it at the time, did what he could to help me bully Mark into letting us address the situation and get paperwork from him that we needed. Eventually we sorted it out, but not without great effort which shouldn't have been necessary, and we deregistered ourselves as a company to prevent such headaches from recurring.

When we finally managed to pin Mark down, he met with me and Simon in a bar in Walthamstow so that we could examine and update the accounts together and start to complete the forms. By then Mark and Simon were both under the auspices of Waltham Forest's 'home treatment team', which aimed in theory to reduce overcrowding on psychiatric wards by providing services normally associated with hospitals, such as medication and contact with nurses, in people's own homes. Home treatment teams were then a recent initiative, based on a dilution of an excellent model developed by the Bradford-based Marxist psychiatrist Pat Bracken, whose pioneering work had highlighted the useful role of service users in steering the work. Hi-jacked by more conventional professionals elsewhere, the user-involvement angle was lost, and the teams became to a large extent simply methods of treating more cheaply people who would otherwise be in hospital. Waltham Forest's version on this occasion involved a social worker arriving at our accounts meeting, having been informed by mobile that Mark and Simon were not at home but in the pub. The social worker sat around looking awkward and nervous for about five minutes as he gave the pair their Olanzipine to wash down with their lager, and watched us preparing accounts and filling in complicated forms the nature of which surely went way over the worker's head.

Southwark Mind's notoriety grew exponentially, and we were attracting grudging respect from within the mainstream mental health field and beyond as one of Britain's leading user-led charities. Projects were developing thick and fast, including a very helpful paperback *Southwark Mental Health Services Directory* compiled by Alex Clark and Sarah Taylor, and a women's group initiated by Jolie Goodman. But the idea of success intimidated some, who still thought that 'user-led' should mean disorganised and downtrodden.

Brian Eageling was a self-styled 'grass roots activist' who had once been involved in a campaign to save mental health users' free bus passes in Lambeth. When I met him he was a chair of Communicate, the nearest the Maudsley hospital had to a patients' council, and he was prominent on the local day centre scene. He also claimed to head MUG, the Maudsley User Group, of which he was the sole member. When Southwark Mind came along he felt threatened and tried to sow divisions within the local user movement, declaring a one-man war on Southwark Mind. A hate mail campaign followed, including several very abusive letters he sent to us with the apparent complicity of Su Glazier, a staff-patient liaison worker employed by the Maudsley who years previously had been instrumental in getting Communicate going. Staff restructuring led to her managers giving her notice to move sideways into a different job, and consciously or unconsciously she seemed to be trying to undermine the group she'd helped create, not wanting to see it function without her.

In the event, she succeeded. Southwark Mind's User Council had offered backing to Communicate to help make their views heard in forums wider than those to which they then had access; Eageling's take on this was to claim, wrongly, that the User Council was undemocratic and trying to take over, submitting draft resolutions for Communicate's meetings attacking Southwark Mind, with Glazier's administrative assistance. I attended one of these meetings, which in the event Eageling failed to attend, and circulated photocopies of some of the vitriolic letters he'd sent us. Communicate members were shocked by the abusive content of the missives, which had tried to imply that Eageling's statements were somehow representative of a constituency which included Communicate members. I also berated Glazier for showing lack of common sense by colluding with the circulation of the divisive material. She pleaded ignorance, in spite of the fact that she'd clearly redrafted many of his mailings, making them reasonably well-written instead of barely literate. The situation illustrated the hostility shown, from some quarters within the user scene, towards user activists perceived as becoming successful: I'd already noticed that Pete Shaughnessy was often treated by other users in the area as if he was a member of staff, rather than a vulnerable person with the courage and ability to make his voice heard, almost entirely on others' behalves.

Eageling's standing fell and Glazier eventually moved sideways within the Maudsley, but Communicate was doomed. The group had for a few years been vocal and inclusive, consisting not only of straightforward psychiatric cases, but also people with drug and alcohol issues using 'dual diagnosis' services based at the Maudsley. Eageling sowed bitter divisions between the two overlapping, as opposed to discrete groups, targeting individuals such as addictions activist Silvio Coutinho. Between them Eageling and Glazier 'edited' Communicate's mailing list, deleting the names of people they disliked with the intention of disenfranchising them from the group's decision-making structure. SIMBA, an acronym for Share in Maudsley Black Action, a new black and minority ethnic user group, was also targeted; and eventually people became so exasperated by the in-fighting that they stopped wanting to be involved, and Communicate stopped happening.

The User Council, once users and professionals alike became accustomed to it, became a successful mechanism by which users influenced how mental health services were developed and delivered. It's often difficult to measure the success of such initiatives because it's hard to tell what services would be like had such groups never existed. For example, staff on psychiatric wards seem less likely to abuse patients' rights if they know that mental health advocates are stalking the hospital, making them less likely to get away with it. The mere existence of user-led scrutiny moderates professional behaviour. We do know that the User Council, during the years I'm referring to, successfully negotiated the prevention of the closure of a popular day centre, the Peckham Pop-in, which was funded by the local mental health trust; and that consultation with local suits took place concerning numerous developments of Southwark's day care services, after-hours services and hospital procedure amongst other things, though we'll never fully know the force of the impact. There were certainly a few failures. Even when we organised a demonstration outside the Maudsley hospital itself, protesting against the cost-cutting closure of some day centres, the closures went ahead regardless. We'd had people chaining themselves to the railings with handcuffs purchased from a sado-masochistic sex shop in Waterloo and received considerable press coverage, but to no avail. What is certain, however, is that such agitation keeps the professionals on their toes, makes them aware that unpopular courses of action will be challenged, and prevents services from deteriorating more than they do anyway.

It was clear too that the high-ranking bureaucrats we were dealing with, senior management from the social services, health authority and trusts, on high wages, were not fundamentally evil people determined to make life as difficult as possible for those who used their services. Most of them seemed to genuinely care and were happy to engage with us, in part because government regulations increasingly gave them a duty to consult, but also because they wished to work out optimum courses of action within the financial restraints imposed on them by the Department of Health. Despite the multi-million pound budgets they oversaw, most of the cash was in fact ring-fenced by the government to support – directly or otherwise – corporate interests. For example, in 2000 the government announced a huge injection of funds into mental health services, but it transpired that most of this money was required by law to be given to pharmaceutical companies via an increase in the NHS psychiatric drugs budget. The spare cash local managers had to play with was minimal. In South East London, millions were squandered on employing agency staff to fill posts which should have been filled by permanent workers, so increasing the rake-off for the private sector; and also on paying for residential facilities outside the borough, increasingly run by the private sector, to contain people with psychiatric diagnoses who had fallen foul of the law and were subject to 'forensic' sections of the mental health act. By law, the bills for such people were footed by the health authorities covering the districts where they were last registered as living. These were generally inner-city boroughs, and many such people were incarcerated for years or even decades, their hope of eventual release dependent on the Home Secretary, and the secure accommodation fees and financial strain in areas such as Lambeth, Southwark and Lewisham were astronomical.

Policy needed to be addressed on a wider than local scale, but Mad Pride rarely engaged with senior government ministers, and when we did it was usually just to wind them up. For example, Pete Shaughnessy took the piss out of former health secretary Frank Dobson during the latter's failed mayoral campaign against Ken Livingstone, in which he polled even less votes than the Tory candidate Steven Norris. We disliked Dobson, because in his former job he'd been the chief parliamentary advocate of coercive and restrictive legislation attacking mental health service users, even describing them as "*nuisance neighbours*" and berating Liberal Democrat MP Simon Hughes for using "*weasel words*" in defence of their civil liberties. Hughes appeared to be the most knowledgeable parliamentarian with regards to mental health issues, and it was interesting that Dobson saw the concept of civil liberties as somehow weasel-like in this context. Civil liberties contradicted his plans to promote the forcible medication of thousands of people in the community, and to lock up further thousands just in case they committed antisocial acts in the future. Clearly, Dobson had it coming.

Livingstone, electioneering, had declared that Dobson was *"clinically depressed"* due to the negative press coverage and public hostility he'd faced during his campaign. Pete issued a press release declaring Mad Pride's support for Dobson, suggesting the slogan *"Mad Frank for Mayor!"* Pete pointed out that we needed respected public figures to come out as mad to help combat stigma and prejudice, and that Dobson would make an inspirational role model for others in similar mental health predicaments. *The Daily Express* and others picked up on this story and it was another nail in Dobson's electoral coffin, as well as being a chance for the roly-poly politician to enjoy what it felt like to be on the receiving end of discrimination. His opponent Livingstone was no angel, and had been subject over the years to numerous accusations of sexual harassment, and off-the-radar corruption allegations involving Gerry Healy's Workers Revolutionary Party and Colonel Gadaffi's Libya which were never reported in the press; but in the event the lesser of the evils prevailed.

Southwark Mind's decision to take on board addictions issues as a serious civil rights concern, even though it had caused controversy at the by now defunct Communicate, once led to an exceptionally good piece of activism involving Silvio Coutinho and a few of his mates carving up a consultation meeting at Cambridge House, where Southwark Mind was based. The local trust, keen to show its commitment to user involvement, was offering ten pounds to anyone who turned up to their 'feedback' and 'sharing information about planning' event. Silvio put the word out, verbally and also using leaflets and posters to the addictions services user community in Southwark and beyond, that all anyone had to do to earn ten pounds was simply to turn up. This led literally to a few hundred street drinkers, heroin addicts and homeless people descending on the meeting with their cans of Tennents Super, causing havoc and preventing any serious consultation from taking place. The trust had only been expecting about twenty people there, which had been the attendance at a recent similar meeting in Lambeth. Some Southwark Mind members were initially furious with Silvio, but I told him immediately that it was one of the finest pieces of activism that I'd ever been privileged to see. This action appeared to demonstrate the need for user consultation within addictions services as well as mental health services, and it led directly to money becoming available to set up an advocacy service, the first of its kind, at the local methadone maintenance clinic.

By the end of 2001, Pete Shaughnessy was starting to lose the plot big time. The attack on the New York twin towers, now known as 9/11, which took place three days before his birthday, had really disturbed him, and he began drinking again after several months on the wagon. He became manic, not for the first time, but with a frightening intensity, and he would never recover from the chain of events this bout of mania set in motion.

My telephone conversations with him had, for several months, been confusing to say the least, with me unable to get a word in edgeways and his conversation skipping uncontrollably from one subject to another. Events at the 2001 Mind annual conference in Scarborough illustrated how distressed he was at the time. He was barely coherent attempting to chat with his mates at the bar, and he had been billed to run a Mad Pride workshop with Simon. Pete ran amok before this could take place. It began when he came across a bearded bartender in the conference centre, and became convinced that this bloke was a member of the Taliban. Pete called him a Taliban cunt and chucked a pint glass at him, showering the beardie with beer and leaving shards and splinters of shattered glass behind. After this Pete stormed out of the centre without looking where he was going, and was nearly run over by a car. *"You cunt!"* Pete shouted at the driver, booting the cunt's car as hard as he could before striding off to the posh hotel where National Mind had booked him a room.

The bar was open late at his hotel and Pete carried on drinking, getting into a series of fights before eventually being carted off by the old bill and spending the night in the local police station. Released without charge, Pete was informed that he was no longer welcome at his hotel. Fortunately, another conference delegate had experienced a similar problem at the hotel he was staying at, so the pair simply swapped rooms. Mind felt it 'inappropriate' for Pete to run the workshop, leaving Simon to facilitate it on his own, with no help from me, as I spent the whole conference in the bar. When it all ended, there were a few hours to kill before the train arrived to take us back to London. Pete had disappeared by then, but several of us decided to visit a hard local Irish republican pub to watch the Republic of Ireland play Iran in a qualifying match that would determine which of the two sides would make it through to the world cup finals the following year. *"Come on you Iranians!"* I shouted drunkenly as I drifted in. Luckily for me, Eddie Murray had been entertaining the regulars with rebel songs previously and he put in a good word for me, probably saving me from being beaten up. Ireland won the match 1-0 and Simon sold some Mad Pride t-shirts.

2002 arrived and it was a bad year. My relationship with Gini was starting to wear me out and Mad Pride had – relatively speaking – fallen into recess. At Southwark Mind I felt for the most part that I was merely treading water, and without the support of some of the excellent workers around me the whole operation might well have collapsed. I was frequently waking up hungover and having panic attacks, and performing the simplest of tasks often felt like wading through treacle. One thing happened that I was pleased with. I'd had an idea that Southwark Mind should produce a manifesto, along the lines of the seminal 1970s manifesto issued by the Campaign Against Psychiatric Oppression but more direct and up to date. With particular help from Alex Clark, the document was developed, articulating what a couple of dozen of us could agree on concerning issues such as the contrasting medical and social models of mental health, what we thought of the police, women's and men's mental health issues, addictions, conditions in hospitals and many more subjects. The manifesto was eventually issued as a paperback book in January 2003.

My powers were waning and my skill at dealing with volatile mad people, which normally I took for granted, decreased with regrettable effects. I was being paid to co-ordinate Southwark Mind and support paid and voluntary staff with severe mental health problems; in fact, much of the time I was receiving as much emotional support from them than I was giving. Unusually for me, I was also blinding myself to some of the increasing tensions between individual staff and management committee members. For example, I was fond of co-chair Sean O'Reilly, who routinely wandered into the offices drunk, and who had a habit of winding people up with verbally aggressive comments which were at times interpreted as sexist. Out of loyalty I tried to defend him, but I was unable to prevent the management committee from kicking him out of Southwark Mind, which made me feel undermined, even though the expulsion was entirely understandable in the circumstances involved. Various staff members were also losing the plot without getting the quality of help from me they might perhaps reasonably have expected.

Southwark Mind's arts collective continued, with outwardly positive results. Sarah Taylor set up a mad art exhibition in a gallery opposite Cambridge House, and on the same day we held a live music and poetry show at Camberwell Jazz Crypt. Such was my confusion at the time that I can't remember for certain who performed at it: the Astronauts may have been involved. Sarah Taylor, a popular and respected worker at Southwark Mind, was herself losing it badly: self-harming, neglecting to eat and being pathologically giving and generous to her own detriment, though she was still functioning at work. I was very worried, and wasn't sure whether to stop her working for the time being, knowing that she wasn't physically up to it, or to let her carry on so as not to further undermine her self-esteem. As it was I simply let things drift. Sarah survived, and went on to set up her own successful mental health arts group Creative Routes. But drift things did, very dangerously, increasingly out of control.

More Trouble Coming Every Day

Ben Watson: *Mad Pride* co-editor, music critic and quasi-academic, once wrote an article about mad music for *The Wire*, a glossy music monthly specialising in arty self-indulgent stuff. It quoted Hugh Metcalfe – organiser of the Klinker, an avant-garde jazz and free improvisation club then running most of its shows in Dalston – criticising Mad Pride, even though he'd never attended any of our events. He felt we were wrong to promote forms of music he considered commercial and that we patronised our audiences by doing so. Mad Pride, he thought, should be more like the Klinker, where musicians played with and in front of each other without a non-participant audience. Although on the whole we liked the Klinker and its performers, we felt that our events should feature acts that people would actually enjoy, and who could draw a crowd and entertain service users, generating a show of strength and helping to draw them into activism surrounding political mental health issues. We didn't mind people being in the audience who weren't going on stage at some point during the show, and this strategy meant that our turnouts always well exceeded single figures, unsettling elitists like Metcalfe. The bands we put on were neither household names nor people experimenting only for their own amusement, but they were people we knew and liked. Metcalfe having raised the issue, Ben, Gini and myself decided to put on a concert featuring some eclectic, avant-garde elements. Ben and Gini decided who the performers would be, and the show was earmarked for November 2002. Significant events took place while the project was in its planning stage.

Penny Shaughnessy, as she was by then known, was becoming understandably exhausted by Pete's mania and confused aggression. Exasperated by Pete's behaviour and the lack of support he and she received from social services and health workers, she kicked him out of their flat in Worthing, after which he travelled around Britain from one town to the next like a silver pellet in a pinball machine. He'd spend a day or so here and there in different places, flitting from police station to psychiatric unit to park bushes, always on the move, resting only to get barred from pubs. No health authority would take any responsibility for him in the districts he visited, their excuse being always that he was registered in Worthing and that staff there should deal with him. Staff in Worthing refused to intervene, because he was not physically within their catchment area.

He was truly mad at this point. He didn't know his arse from his elbow. Exhausted but still manic, he turned up on my doorstep one night in September 2002 and stayed in my flat for a month. I tried to look after him as best I could, but other pressures meant that I was spreading myself too thinly. Gini had recently moved into a mortgaged flat and wanted support and company there: she thought I should *"get my priorities right"*. I was still paid to run Southwark Mind, where a larger than usual proportion of my friends and colleagues were themselves unwell. There seemed to be too many priorities, my own well-being least among them.

I knew all about the terrible things attached to the sharp end of psychiatric services: the incarceration and loss of liberty, the coercion and forced medication, the arrogant doctors not listening, the boredom, the stigma and the tasteless hospital food. Nevertheless I attempted to persuade Pete to go to hospital, in the absence of any better alternatives, and concerned for Pete's safety. His behaviour at the time was outrageously bizarre, and sometimes funny, as when he found a double-decker bus with the keys in the ignition at London Bridge station, hi-jacked it and drove it all the way to Worthing, where he parked it outside a psychiatric emergency clinic. After waiting several hours for a doctor who never came, he became bored and drove the bus back to London Bridge before walking back to my flat. More disturbingly, he was habitually going into pubs, although by this stage he was on the wagon, and he would provoke arguments and fights apparently on some self-harm trip, in the hope of being beaten up. He was experiencing life as if it was something he was dreaming. Very few people really feel like using services when they're manic, worried that the fun will be made to stop, though Pete's deluded and dangerous behaviour clearly wasn't much fun. Pete, who knew exactly what went on in hospitals, was understandably reluctant to seek help. His moments of wishing to co-operate with services were fleeting, and my efforts – unsupported by Pete's other friends who were either exasperated or out of their depth – failed. True to my principles, I didn't entertain the idea of getting him sectioned by summoning either the police or social workers on the grounds of urgent high risk, without warning him. This would have been the only way he'd have received help at this stage, but rightly or wrongly I thought this would amount to a breach of trust.

It didn't help that I was at Gini's place most nights as she was allergic to my cats Magic and Grey One, in any case unhappy to visit my place and unwilling to be left alone, leaving Pete in my flat by himself much of the time. My neighbours, realising that he was insane, thought I was negligent for leaving him on his own, and they were right. They became scared of Pete wandering loose around the block of flats and involving them in strange conversations about his esoteric plans to take over the government of Nigeria in order to sort out the entire continent of Africa. With Pete's permission, I called his key worker a few times in Pete's official town of residence, Worthing. *"What the fuck am I supposed to do about it?"* the sympathetic worker may as well have said. *"He's in London now!"* If he'd been any good, he'd have sent a team up from Worthing to my flat to assess Pete.

The crunch came when Pete lost his key and arrived back at three o'clock in the morning when I was out. Pete broke into a school for special needs kids behind the flats, and stole two ladders. Carrying these, he climbed over a few fences and through various back gardens until he was at the back of the block, where he used the ladders to get in through a window I'd left unlocked, leaving them propped against the wall outside. The neighbours felt still more unsettled by this, and there were hints that they were considering obtaining a court injunction banning Pete, and possibly me, from the building. I explained to Pete that he needed to leave. Somewhere through the madness this registered and he went off, had a fight and was sectioned almost immediately.

When he came out of hospital he was clearly very depressed and lacking in confidence. He'd lost a lot of weight and was staying with his dad in Dulwich. After his protracted spell of mania he'd come right down and it was unimaginably hard for him. He realised that he'd fucked up his marriage to Penny, possibly irreparably, and he wasn't looking forward to trying to pick up the pieces after the madness. He was as sensitive and articulate as we knew him to be at his best, but he was struggling and in terrible pain. Complacently, Pete's friends – including me – behaved as if he'd be all right, trying to believe that his reputation as a pillar of strength would overcome everything. He was let out in time to attend a demonstration on 14th September 2002, his fortieth birthday. The so-called 'Mental Health Alliance', consisting of several mental health charities including Mind, Rethink, and even SANE who by then were pretending to go along with the consensus of informed opinion for fear of becoming marginalised, had called for a march from Whitehall to the Imperial War Museum, site of the original Bedlam, to oppose the continuing threat of community treatment orders to allow shrinks to forcibly medicate anyone, anytime. While the demo was being organised, a young girl was murdered in Soham, out in the sticks to the south-west of London, by a man who had never been anywhere near any mental health services, but whose state of mind was instantly subject to intense media speculation, reinforcing the public's suspicion of those labelled mentally ill. Stupidly, the 'alliance' cancelled the demo, worrying that it could backfire in the context of the Soham murder. Mind tried to cover itself by issuing a statement, claiming that they disagreed with the cancellation and in an ideal world would have gone ahead with the protest anyway, but unfortunately they couldn't find enough stewards at such short notice.

Unimpressed by this collective sell-out by proper professionals from mainstream charities, service users across the UK decided that they didn't need permission from the charities to demonstrate and that the protest would take place regardless. In particular a group from Brighton calling themselves No Force took the lead: networking, spreading publicity and making props in only a few short days without concerning themselves about any perceived need for stewards. A great deal of people were confused by the mixed messages now appearing about whether the demo would actually happen, making the turnout far smaller than it could have been. Nevertheless, nearly a thousand of us turned up, and there was hardly a professional in sight.

We gathered at Whitehall and user groups from all over Britain swapped leaflets, newsletters and information. We handed out pamphlets printed specifically for the demo to ordinary members of the public as we marched past them, and far from encountering hostility as the Mental Health Alliance had feared, the response we received was overwhelmingly encouraging. Even as we chanted the co-opted Millwall slogan, *"we are mental, we are evil, no one likes us, we don't care"*, normals who we happened to pass cheered and stuck their thumbs up at us. Ian Spikey Thing's samba band came along and sounded especially loud when their bongos echoed beneath a railway bridge at Waterloo. Marching past Downing Street, service users were shouting out 'wankers!' and 'cunts!' in unison and making appropriate gestures; and that notorious symbol of authority, Big Ben, also came in for some verbal abuse. Finally we arrived at the War Museum, where several activists, including user psychologist Dr Rufus May who was beginning to make a name for himself in the media, Lynne Clayton, and even me gave speeches using a cheap hand-held megaphone. Most people know the drill when marches come to an end: it involves milling around for about an hour while spokespeople harangue. And then we went off to the pub. Here I chatted to Pete, Gini, Ben, and others, including Danielle Rosier from the local SWP. She'd been sent to review the demo for the party's fanzine, *Socialist Worker*, and she was on enforced gardening leave from her job at the home office, where she'd been labelled crazy. She seemed like a potentially useful person to know.

Around this time, I had acute pancreatitis again and ended up in hospital. Gini was very supportive, and Julie Hathaway was simultaneously on a psychiatric ward in a nearby block so I had people to talk to, but still became very bored when I started to feel a bit better after a few days, wandering around the corridors aimlessly by day and feeling agitated and sleepless all night whilst attached to those transparent tubes and a seven-feet tall t-shaped metal thing with wheels on. The hospital wanted to keep me in for a few weeks ostensibly to be on the safe side, but I interpreted this suggestion as a punishment for being self-inflictedly ill, and I planned my escape route. Treatment for pancreatitis itself felt like a punishment, involving the 'nil by mouth' routine whereby I wasn't allowed to eat or drink at all for a few days, and different doctors would give conflicting messages about when I could start eating again, confusing the nurses. I'd had enough. At Homerton hospital the drunks being treated for alcohol-related diseases, in other words half of all of the patients, had to congregate in the only part of the building where smoking was allowed: a designated stairwell which had nicotine-yellowed walls and ceilings, a permanent carpet of empty cans of Tennents Super and used needles, and a few benches on which local homeless junkies slept illicitly at night. A spirit of comradeship was ever-present in the stairwell, and the other drunks created a diversion to assist me in escaping through the back entrance when the nurses weren't looking. Once outside I ran like fuck, with plastic things still inserted into my veins after I'd ripped the tubes out. Manually getting these out wasn't easy and I had to self-treat an infection afterwards, but I'm sure I got better a lot more quickly on the outside than I would have done if I'd remained in hospital.

Jason Pegler, Sean O'Reilly and myself were booked in to deliver a lecture about 'creativity and recovery' at 2002's three-day Mind Annual Conference in Cardiff. The conference had a theme around recovery, which was the latest buzzword. We'd thought about calling the lecture 'recovery, why bother?' but figured the conference organisers wouldn't be too keen on this. Jason, a young author, had published a racy autobiography *A Can of Madness*, a uniquely egotistical account of his experiences of 'manic depression', as it was called before being re-branded 'bipolar disorder'. He'd also set up a vanity paperback imprint, Chipmunkapublishing, specialising in mad memoirs by various other authors, the most talented of them being South London's Dolly Sen. Mind annual conferences were a good excuse for Southwark Mind folks to stay in a smart hotel and get pissed with other mental health bores from all over Britain: and in fact, the important connections were always made not in workshops or lectures, which could vary from groundbreakingly useful to embarrassingly dull, but in the bars. I'd first met Jason at a previous conference and he'd been talking about his plans to publish his autobiography. Cynically, I assumed that he'd never get it together, and that if he did the book would be useless anyway. In fact, it was pretty good: a raw, candid and at times unintentionally hilarious account full of outrageous boasts and compulsive, lucid energy. Jason always wore a smart suit and tie and had mastered the language used by business people, which helped him to set up a series of scams. We arranged a few meetings to prepare the lecture, but Sean failed to turn up to any of them and seemed to have disappeared from the face of the earth, so we recruited Ben Watson to replace him. On the first day of the conference as I stood on a platform with a dozen or so Southwark Mind activists waiting for the train to take us to Cardiff, Sean rang me on my mobile, very drunk, expecting to come along. I was surprised he'd remembered it, but he gave me quite a mouthful when I explained to him that Ben had stepped in. It wasn't the last mouthful that I received during those three days.

Miles, an ex-boyfriend of Gini and former member of South London avant-garde band Bourbonese Quark, had hung himself a few days earlier in his flat in the Heygate estate, Elephant and Castle. His life over the previous few years had been a sharp downward spiral into heroin addiction, for which Gini partly and I think mistakenly held herself responsible, and he'd run out of friends, possessions and self-respect. I accompanied Gini when she went to identify the body on the following day. Understandably she was very distressed, almost to the point of psychosis, and frequently kept me up all night ranting, repetitively deflecting her grief onto people not directly involved, under the influence of copious quantities of cocaine and vodka. It was hard work, I was exhausted, and continuing to work at Southwark Mind full time was becoming ever more difficult. The funeral took place midway through the Mind conference. The day before I went to Cardiff, Gini attempted to kill a couple of passers-by. Two Turkish guys were blocking her path as she turned a corner in her car to approach her home, forcing her to brake. After she shouted abuse at them they gave her a funny look, which convinced her that they deserved the death penalty: someone had to pay for Miles' suicide and the Turks had asked for it. Screaming, she reversed her motor and was about to ram the fuckers into a brick wall when I opened the passenger seat door and jumped out, not entirely convinced that she was choosing the correct course of action. This made her redirect her anger towards me, letting the Turks off the hook. Sensibly, I ran up an alleyway too small for her car to follow as she hurled incoherent insults in my direction. She parked her car and went into her flat, and I followed after giving her time to cool off a little. Angrily, she accused me of disloyalty for failing to support her murder mission, and made it clear that she didn't want me around over the period of Miles' funeral, which in any case she thought inappropriate for me to attend.

I wasn't sure whether to take her at her word, but felt responsible for helping the gang of South London lunatics to their hotel in Cardiff in one piece, figuring that Gini would have other friends to keep an eye on her. In any case I was supposed to deliver a lecture with Jason and Ben. My comrades at Southwark Mind had been more supportive and tolerant of me than I could reasonably have expected during the previous, difficult few months, and I felt under an obligation to try to keep the work together, but the train ride there was a minor fiasco. Pete Shaughnessy was expelled from the train at one of the stations along the route for calling another passenger a cunt and nearly provoking a fight; he had to wait for the next train in order to complete his journey. I sat with a group of other seasoned drinkers, there being plenty of us at Southwark Mind, and we shared the bottle of whiskey Chris Matheson had brought with him and cleaned the buffet car out of lager. When we arrived at the hotel a number of us were intoxicated, making the rest of our crew nervous, sensing trouble ahead. I went upstairs to my room and attempted to sober up with coffee. We'd all arranged to meet at seven o'clock to go out for a corporate meal, for which my presence was vital, because I had the cheque book. As I came back downstairs my mobile went off, and it was Gini shouting very loud, fast and angrily, aggrieved that I'd ventured all the way to Cardiff leaving her to face Miles' funeral without me. Simultaneously, as I sat beside a public hotel telephone, Les Elliott from Southwark Mind approached shouting rather insistently that I was late, and that people were hungry. And they obviously were. Gini was shouting into one ear, Southwark Mind into the other. Feeling rattled and still drunk, I told Les to fuck off, and he seemed to get the message. Soon after Gini rang off and Southwark Mind went to look for somewhere to eat. None of us knew Cardiff and it took a while to find a suitable place, which some of the crew seemed to think was my fault, and they became bad-tempered. As we were about to enter the pizza place that we finally chose, Gini rang again and stupidly I answered, allowing myself to be harangued further. I sat in a doorway holding the phone to my ear, provoking a gang of Southwark Mind to tell me to hang up and get the fuck on with it. They were hungry. *"Fuck off, the lot of you!"* I shouted, chucking the handset aggressively at a bin. It was the first time I'd lost my temper since the row with Debbie McNamara in Pumpkins two years earlier. The phone was broken. We went inside and I felt awkward so I went off to a nearby pub, leaving the others to eat, returning in time to pay the bill.

The next day was the eve of Miles' funeral, and by way of compromise I'd decided to go back to London, and then return a day later to Cardiff in time for the lecture on the morning of the last day of the conference. Gini had calmed down a little and composed a speech for the funeral, also running it past me: she was still in shellshock with grief. Back in Wales by the following evening, I drank through the night with Simon Morris from Ceramic Hobs, Ben Watson, Shirley Pearson, Chris Matheson and a few other shady characters. Through the haze it appeared that we had less hotel rooms between us than we thought we'd had, but I managed to grab a couple of hours' kip on Chris's floor.

While I'd been back in London to help keep Gini calm, Southwark Mind members had organised a protest at a mass 'plenary' meeting in the main Cardiff conference centre hall. A Labour health minister was speaking, trying to defend the government's proposed mental health bill which included the hated community treatment orders. Led by Cath Collins, a gang of service users – Pete Shaughnessy among them – invaded the stage during the politician's speech waving placards with slogans such as 'No Force', 'No to Community Treatment Orders' and 'Zito is Wrong'. National Mind had always claimed not to like community treatment orders either but nevertheless as usual they were unhappy with the confrontational approach emanating from South East London.

Remarkably, given the 23 pints of lager he'd consumed the day before, Chris was bright and bubbly in the morning, managing to wake me up in time for the lecture and even giving me some of his valium to control the shakes. Arriving at the lecture hall, I discovered that indoor smoking was banned and that Pete Shaughnessy had set up a merchandise stall in front of the Mad Pride banner. Me, Ben and Jason sat behind a desk armed with a microphone and got on with the show. After years working in London with Mad Pride and Southwark Mind, both broad-minded groups, I'd forgotten how conservative service users from the sticks could be. The hundred or so folks in the audience consisted almost entirely of users from far-flung corners, and I began by announcing: "*We're* Mad Pride! *We don't take any notice of rules and regulations, so we can all snout up in here!*" The mad bumpkins responded by looking uncomfortable and staring nervously at their shoes.

Figuring that perhaps we should tone things down a little I chose to nip out to the toilets whenever I wanted a fag during the lecture, but apparently this moderation wasn't sufficient to keep the conservatives happy. Jason kicked off the show, nervous and ill-prepared, and after giving a faltering speech he couldn't decide which passage of *A Can of Madness* to read. I directed him to a chapter in his book where he has a delusion in which he's shagging all five of the Spice Girls one by one in a shower, and he recited this passage. A few London Mad Pride groupies tittered appreciatively, but the majority of the crowd was unimpressed. Then, after giving some spiel about the relationship between madness and rebel creativity, I offered to verbally deliver one of the sex scenes from *Seaton Point*, but I was shouted down by people scared of being offended. Instead I recited an equally unpleasant scene involving a difficult vampire childbirth, which made the audience even more hostile. Ben was next, slagging off Survivors Poetry for being too mainstream and for daring to promote poets who simply weren't any good. He followed his speech with one of his own epic avant-garde poems which, typically, made no conventional sense, provoking onlookers to question why he wasn't writing directly about his own personal experience. His use of the word 'cunt' in his work also had people glaring spitefully, probably concerned for his hell-bound soul. Finally, after a question and answer slot, we showed Gini's video of Ceramic Hobs' 'Make Mine a Large One', during which half of the mad yokels walked out in protest, shouting 'disgusting!' in a collective display of righteous indignation. We weren't invited back to speak at any further Mind annual conferences, and in the subsequent book issued by Mind about the Cardiff get-together, all references to our lecture were accompanied by a corporate disclaimer.

The show that me, Ben and Gini had been planning was billed as 'Down With the Mental Health Bill!' and it took place at the Bull and Gate, Kentish Town, a week after the conference. It was heavily promoted, and the venue was sold out. The nine acts included live artist friends of Gini performing some strange visual pieces, and various avant-garde improvisation friends of Ben making a holy racket. I was master of ceremonies, and the show as a whole was edgy and celebratory. Gini's Ceramic Hobs video was shown and went down much better than it had in Cardiff. When I described from the stage how it had been received by the mad inbreds in Wales, audience members shouted that it was *"not disgusting enough"*, proving that London is cooler than the sticks. Other highlights came from country-rocker Alan Tyler; Mat Fraser, the short-armed actor and disability rights media spokesperson singing some thalidomide disco numbers; and, most notably, Jim MacDougall's punk band Apeshit who by then had already released ten full-length albums on CD.

Jim MacDougall lived his entire life as one big performance art piece. He was in the habit of wandering around London armed with a hidden minidisk machine, provoking altercations with members of the public, recording the results and then releasing them on his albums. He was awaiting trial for setting fireworks off on the tube, a situation which would lead to a short prison sentence in Pentonville, and his many previous scrapes with the old bill had included being found guilty of a bomb hoax, leading to months in a secure unit for the criminally insane. I'd been the intended recipient of one of the packages labelled *"caution: letter bomb enclosed"* left at Homerton High Street post office, but sadly the missive never reached me, and was instead confiscated by the police who failed to see the funny side: in fact they evacuated a half-mile portion of Homerton. Years back, Jim had published *My Catholic Enemy*, a magazine of short stories used as a vehicle for violence, blasphemy, unpleasant pornography and anything else offensive he could think of. Realising that Jim spent a lot of time at the Hackney charity Core Arts, a local attention-seeker and troublemaker named Heather Beveridge had gone through the magazine with a yellow marker pen highlighting the best bits, and shown them out of context to various funders and other people she thought might help cause problems, and Core Arts was threatened with losing some of its funding. My take on this was simply to reprint some of the more outrageous extracts in the Mad Pride anthology, provoking Beveridge to waste weeks wandering around London arguing with people who worked in book shops, trying unsuccessfully to persuade them to remove the book from their shelves. She'd turned up at the Mad Pride

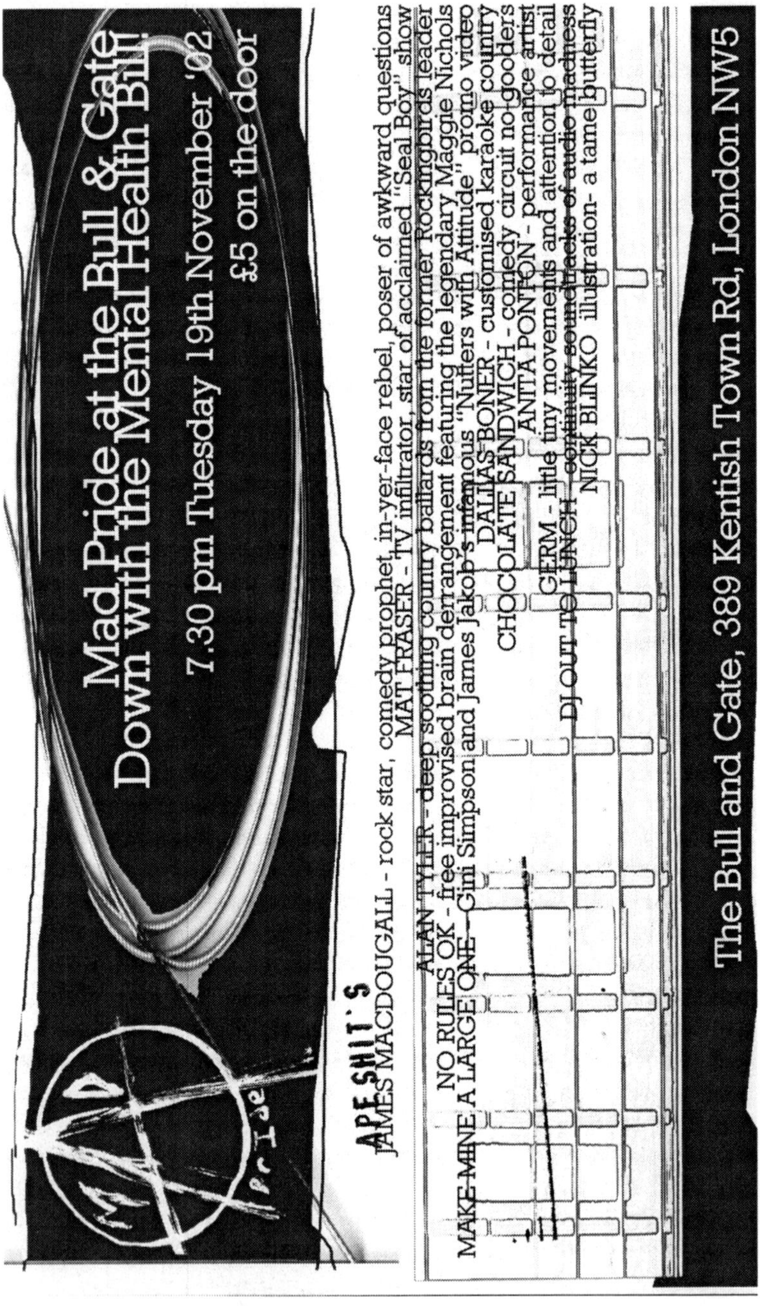
Mad Pride at the Bull & Gate
Down with the Mental Health Bill!
7.30 pm Tuesday 19th November '02
£5 on the door
APESHIT'S
JAMES MACDOUGALL - rock star, comedy prophet, in-yer-face rebel, poser of awkward questions
MAT FRASER - TV infiltrator, star of acclaimed "Seal Boy" show
ALAN TYLER - deep soothing country ballards from the former Rockingbirds leader
NO RULES OK - free improvised brain derrangement featuring the legendary Maggie Nichols
MAKE MINE A LARGE ONE - Gini Simpson and James Jakob's infamous "Nutters with Attitude" promo video
DALLAS BONER - customised karaoke country
CHOCOLATE SANDWICH - comedy circuit no-gooders
ANITA PONTON - performance artist
GERM - little tiny movements and attention to detail
DJ OUT TO LUNCH - continuity soundtracks of audio madness
NICK BLINKO illustration- a tame butterfly
The Bull and Gate, 389 Kentish Town Rd, London NW5

festival in Clissold Park, and had been aggrieved that I wouldn't let her read any of her poems from the stage I'd been managing, on the grounds that I disliked her. On that occasion she'd retaliated by threatening to report us to our funders for various imagined crimes; she was disappointed when I pointed out to her that we didn't have any funders. By way of contrast Jim was one of the good guys, and at the Mad Pride show at the Bull and Gate he had a respectful and appreciative audience who lovingly threw cans, bottles and rolled up pieces of paper at him as he sang his cutting-edge semi-improvised punk songs backed by some great musicians from Core Arts. The concert as a whole was an unqualified triumph. For Pete Shaughnessy standing quietly behind a merchandise stall, it was the last live show he would ever attend.

On December 14th 2002, Alternative TV performed at the Dublin Castle in Camden. Midway through their set their drummer needed to take a piss. Simon Barnett, who had escaped for the evening from the psychiatric ward on which he was by then incarcerated, decided to deputise during a rendition of 'The Force is Blind'. He'd never played drums before in his life, but the performance still ended up on a live album. He was looking forward to telling Pete about his moment of rock'n'roll stardom, but he never had the chance.

On December 15th 2002, Pete chucked himself under a train at Battersea station. Cath Collins, who heard the news before me, phoned me at Southwark Mind's offices the following day and shared the news. It was my 38th birthday. I'd arranged to go to Tadims, a Turkish café in Camberwell, to celebrate with a few Southwark Mind characters and others. This went ahead, a gang of us crying into cheap Turkish red wine that tasted like rancid vinegar. Tuba Karacalar managed to get me into a taxi home in one piece. At the time, Barbara, Nikki Sudden's girlfriend, was living in the spare room in my flat because she was working on a placement with Vivienne Westwood as part of a fashion design degree course. Barbara seemed quite straight, and at times I wondered if she found the severe chaos and dissolution evident in the flat to be troublesome and alien. Whenever I had such thoughts, I had to remind myself that she'd been going out with Nikki Sudden for five years, disproving this theory. Nikki often stayed there, as on this occasion, and when I let myself in it seemed strange that he was wishing me a happy birthday in his usual cheerful manner. He didn't have too long to go either.

Pete's funeral was on Christmas Eve. He'd telephoned me a week before his death, in what had appeared to be an unusually earnest frame of mind. He told me that he'd never felt so depressed before: coming from him, this was saying something very extreme. I made him promise not to take any rash actions. Promises, promises. The call lasted for at least half an hour, and we shared feelings of mutual love and respect for each other. It didn't then seriously occur to me that he was saying goodbye.

Gini, Frank Bangay, Hugh Mulhall and me shared a taxi from Hackney to East Dulwich in Southwark in time for the service, at the unearthly hour of half past nine in the morning. Gini was still very much in a traumatised state of grief after what had happened to Miles. Pete was the latest in a long line of friends for both of us who had died young: almost all of them by suicide or drug overdoses. It felt as if death was all there was, but I don't think I'd ever felt as badly affected by someone's demise before. I'd known Pete for a little less than five years, but it felt as if we'd fought in a war together, side by side in the trenches. It all seemed empty and unreal, and it was as if the previous five years hadn't really happened but were just part of some hallucinatory fantasy occurring as a reward for taking too much acid back when I was a teenager. The fact was that these five years had led to this funeral.

Four hundred people were there. Some of them were respectable professional characters like Simon Hughes from the Liberal Democrats who, despite being a politician and a Liberal Democrat, had always been nice to us. Isobel Morris, senior services manager at the Maudsley, had turned up and looked as upset as anyone else: Pete had always had this skill of attracting not even grudging admiration from establishment figures who were frequently on the receiving end of his campaigning and pranks. Such successful people were used to being out of bed by half past nine, unlike the rest of the doubly disorientated mourners: football fans Pete had known through his association with Dulwich Hamlet FC; anarchists and anti-globalisation activists, many of them from Brighton and Worthing; an array of relatives from Pete's extended Irish family; and an enormous turnout of mental health service users. Some of us were high-profile campaigners and troublemakers. Others were people who struggled simply to stay alive, the limits of whose ambitions went no further than the nearest day centre; who felt grateful when their basic needs were met, if they were lucky enough to have a roof over their heads on one impoverished council estate or other; people whose most urgent worry was sometimes whether the DLA renewal application form every couple of years or so would be successful, determining whether they'd have enough to eat in the foreseeable future; people who faced daily battles with prejudiced neighbours who they struggled to communicate with, and who may or may not have been pissed off with the noise coming out of their flats; people who felt scared of mental health professionals who had not learnt how to listen; people troubled by physically debilitating side effects of anti-psychotic medication, as well as the debilitation caused by the mental health conditions themselves, and also the loneliness, boredom, poverty and alienation, the unpredictable but ubiquitous threats issued from a society that didn't give a fuck. And it was for these people, for the quality of their lives, that Pete had had the audacity to ask for more, putting his head above the parapet and demanding respect, even as the bullets flew around him. Many of the users at the funeral knew very little of the work that Pete had done to promote the civil liberties and social standing of those labelled mad. All they knew was that he was a good bloke, always kind, generous, thoughtful and funny, who had hung around mental health services and who had always and in any situation, even at his most crazy, somehow managed to have some kind of leadership role conferred upon him.

There was a ceremony, with a priest uttering some hocus pocus which made the hard-core Catholics in Pete's family feel better, and giving a resume of Pete's life which totally overlooked the controversial stuff that had made him famous. Pete's father was still alive and had become accustomed to close family members' funerals. Some years before, one of Pete's sisters had been murdered in a knife attack by a boyfriend later labelled with schizophrenia and sent to a special hospital. This had been one of the defining events of Pete's life. Instead of reacting like Jayne Zito, who had demanded that people whose mental health was fragile should be locked up to minimise risks to normal people, Pete wanted to understand what lay behind such horror, seeing no reason why pursuit of vengeance directed either at the killer or deflected onto a community of service users as a whole would help anyone. There was nothing ironic about the fact that this attitude led him to become one of the most effective campaigners for mad peoples' rights that this country has ever seen. It was entirely rational that he took his anguish and anger out not on his sister's killer, who Pete thought was simply yet another victim, but on an insane capitalist system which, through its various branches including mainstream psychiatry, is at the root of so much of this tragedy. Pete even, for a time, worked as a mental health advocate at Broadmoor, the exact place where his sister's killer was incarcerated.

Pete had always said that, should he predecease his father, he'd like to be buried in order to keep the old man happy; otherwise, he wanted to be cremated. In the event, Pete was buried on the same plot as his sister and his mum, and was joined there by his dad a little later. At the burial, Simon and I tied the original Mad Pride banner, a spray-painted bed sheet I'd designed the night before the first Mad Pride show, to the railings opposite the plot. And then we left it there, fluttering in the wind, and left Pete there, in the ground, taken from us way too soon. After this we went to the wake, where Eddie Murray performed some songs including John Lennon's somehow appropriate 'Working Class Hero'. And then we went to Penny's mum's nearby flat and continued to drown our sorrows. We fantasised late in the evening about going to Battersea train station there and then to trash it in revenge: after all, the place had it coming; but in fact our fight had left us by then. Christmas, for that year, was cancelled.

I'd been thinking about blowing out my job at Southwark Mind, aware of my declining ability to hack it properly, and Pete's death was the last straw. I gave notice, telling my comrades there that I'd finish in February 2003. The exhaustion of my reserves of physical and emotional energy and what remained of my nerves was the excuse I needed to retire from wage slavery.

On January 4th, Southwark Mind's Arts Collective held a 'Beat the New Year Blues' show at Camberwell Jazz Crypt, with performances by some local mad poets and musicians. Handily, Nikki Sudden was still resident in my flat, and was available for an acoustic set singing his songs of everyday substance misuse, romantic misadventure and self-injury. Most mental health charities wouldn't have wanted someone like Nikki performing in front of their clients. They'd have been worried that he'd lead them astray. Fortunately, Southwark Mind wasn't like most

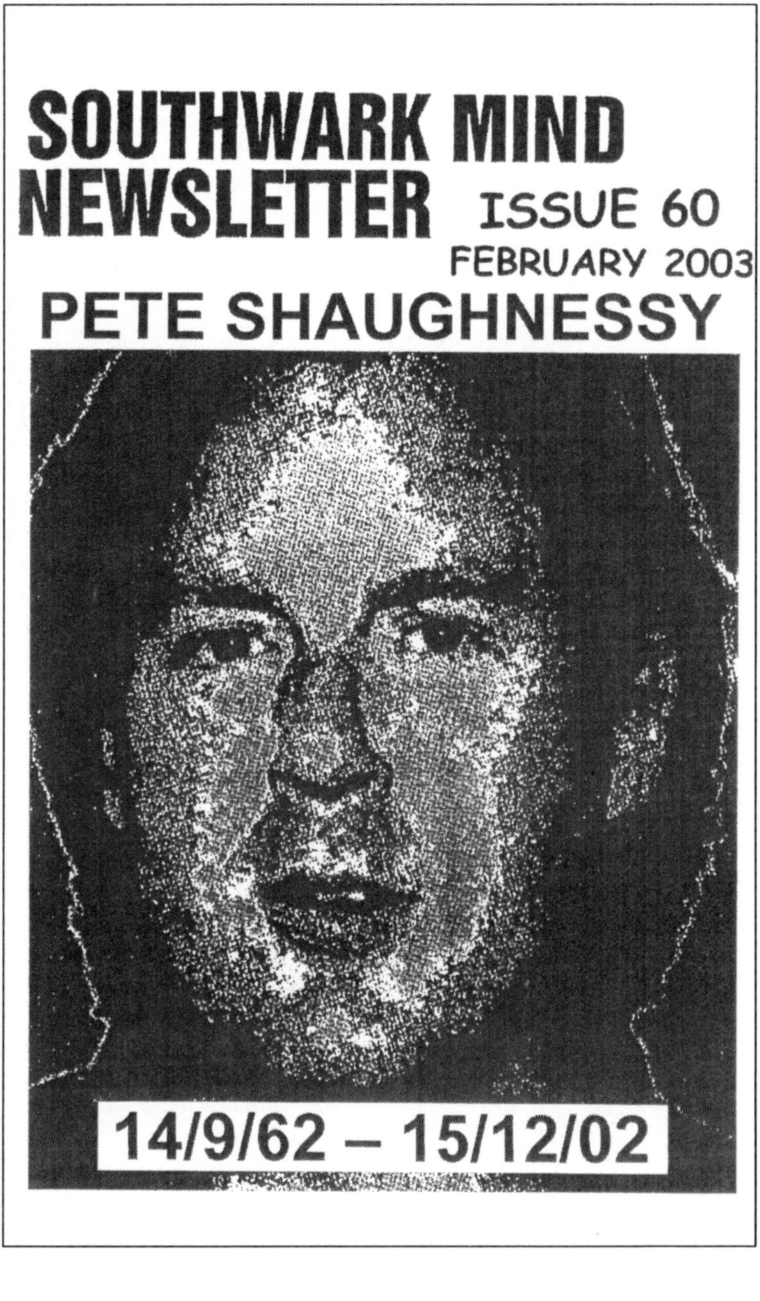
SOUTHWARK MIND
NEWSLETTER
ISSUE 60
FEBRUARY 2003
PETE SHAUGHNESSY
14/9/62 – 15/12/02

charities, and the majority of us had led ourselves astray already. Because it was a quiet week, *the Guardian* made the show a pick of the week in their rock and pop listings. It had been ages since Nikki had more than a cult following in Britain, but a fair few foreign tourists turned up, and they were confused to find themselves in a situation which more resembled a psychiatric ward with a bar in it than a typical rock event. My supervisor Rick Henderson had just formed a punk trio called Arnie, and they performed their debut show; Frank Bangay, Jim MacDougall and Tony Palfrey also performed. Less than three weeks after Pete's death, the show felt strangely unreal to me, but the vibe was as celebratory as could have been expected in the circumstances.

Issue #60 of *Southwark Mind Newsletter* came out at the beginning of February: 28 pages of tributes and grief. Dozens of Pete's friends and fans contributed their reactions and recollections: doctors, journalists, rock stars, charity bosses, and most importantly, rank and file mental health service users from South London all had their tales to share. I've no idea how I managed to get this magazine together given the state I was in, so quickly and so soon after the event. I gather that Danielle Rosier typed and designed some of it. I've no recollection of any of it, but it was the best single issue of a magazine I'd ever helped produce, full of unbelievable intensity and power: a fitting tribute. Pete's chapter from the Mad Pride anthology was reprinted in the newsletter, and it was probably the most intense contribution of them all. Its penultimate paragraph described a conversation Pete had held with a suicidal ex-girlfriend who had been abused as a child in a children's home. *"Hand on heart,"* Pete wrote, *"she's probably better off where she is now"*.

Pete didn't get things right every time and he hadn't then. But there was no arguing with the final paragraph. *"I see life as one big swimming pool. Some of us are thrust into the deep end and we manage to survive. We make our way down to the shallow end, where it's easy, boring. The people there are scared of the deep end, scared of the unknown, so they shun people like me and call me MAD. Madness is a natural reaction. The worker who abused Louise at six years old is the killer."*

Southwark Mind's manifesto was released as a paperback around the same time, summarising what we could all agree on regarding issues relating to mental health and its treatment. The manifesto and issue #60 of the magazine were a good way for

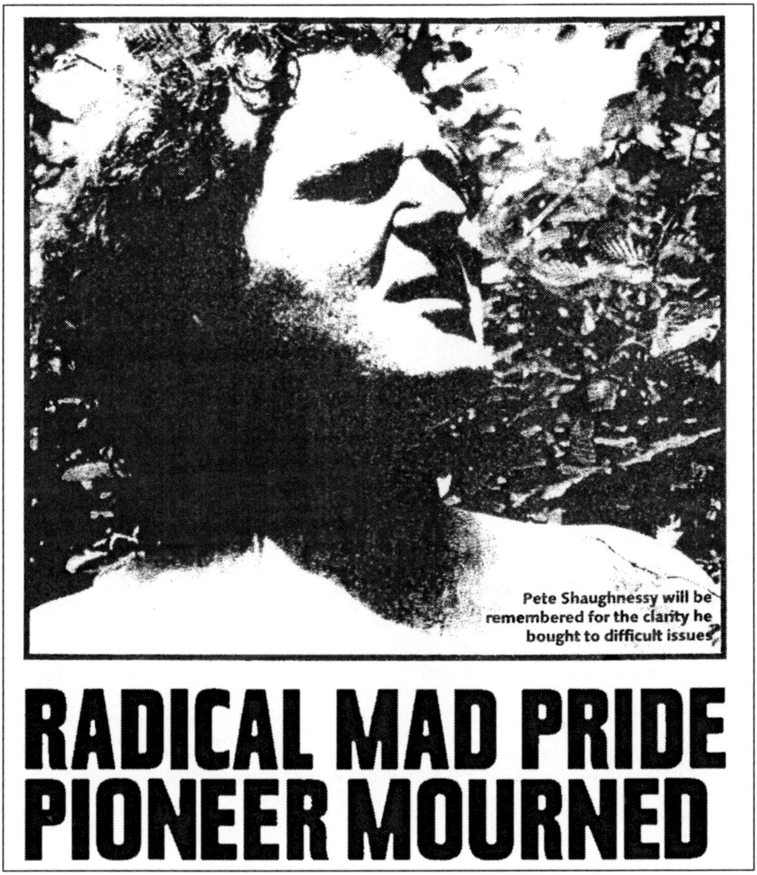
Pete Shaughnessy will be remembered for the clarity he bought to difficult issues

RADICAL MAD PRIDE PIONEER MOURNED

Pete Shaughnessy obituary, The Big Issue

me to round things up before being told, nicely, to leave a few days before the notice that I'd given was due to expire. At the time the manifesto was perceived by many as being 'that lot up to their usual tricks', radical gesture politics that would simply lose friends and alienate people. Most of its contents now are representative of consensual opinion within the mental health user movement. But as it has been with most of the significant activity emanating from Southwark Mind, Mad Pride, and before that the Hackney Advocacy Service, my friends and myself have been remembered neither for our innovations, nor for the development of service models and ways of understanding mental health issues which, had we patented them, would mean

SIMON BARNETT FROM MAD PRIDE WRITES...

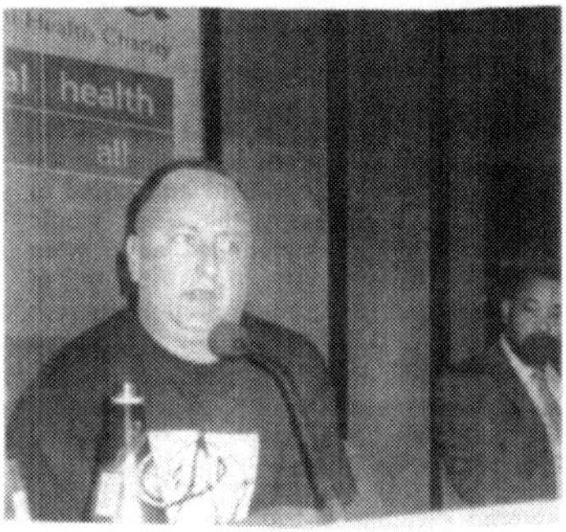

This has to be the most difficult thing I've ever written. Pete Shaughnessy, a great man and true friend is dead. The last month has been a daze. Christmas and new year have passed, seemingly everybody rushing around enjoying themselves, whilst I've been feeling anger and extreme sadness, then shock and disbelief.

I'm sure Newsletter readers will know about Pete's vision, hard work and skills that have made Southwark Mind almost unique as a service user-managed and staffed organisation, but I've been trying to think of something different and personal to say. The joy of Pete's funeral and wake was to see so many people there. This confirmed how popular Pete was, how much he got around, and just how many peoples' lives he touched.

I first met Pete at the Justice for the Liverpool Dockers march in about 1996. At the time I was running a Manic Depression Fellowship group in Waltham Forest. The woman I was with happily cried "it's Pete!" and went running up. Pete was apparently running an MDF group in South London at the time. We were introduced. He was coolly standing at the side of the road, basking at the sun: it was if he was watching, thinking he could organise something similar connected to mental health.

Of course, that's what he did. Lots of other people helped, but I always found Pete inspirational. I honestly believe that without Reclaim Bedlam, Pete's brainchild, there would be no Mad Pride. Mad Pride was conceived in a manic rant but Pete kept the idea going and introduced me to so many other people without whom we would never have achieved what we have.

For me, Pete took grass-roots mental health issues into the media in a new and exciting way. I'm not dismissing the bravery of people who had told their life stories to the press before; however, TV coverage of the campaigning work was somehow much more exciting.

I'll miss Pete, a lot. I'll miss those long telephone conversations with his voice croaking, probably from smoking and talking so much. Those conversations were enlightening on topics such as politics, non-league football and Irish history, and life in general. He was very funny and insightful.

But his tenderness was beautiful as well. On the steps of St. Paul's Cathedral at the commemorative picket, I was agitated, upset, a little manic even. With a few words Pete calmed me.

My heartfelt sympathy goes to Penny, his children, his family and all his friends locally and nationally. Rest in peace, Peter Anthony Shaughnessy.

Pete Shaughnessy obituary by Simon Barnett, Southward MIND news

that we'd never have to work again. We're remembered instead mostly for the controversy our ideas – and the ways in which we put them across – generated at the time, and our reputations as troublemakers will always follow us and trip us up.

It was nice, for a while afterwards, to have the opportunity to sit in the pub all day, feeling miserable on my own with no-one interfering. But escape wasn't a realistic expectation because I was taking myself with me wherever I went, which for a while wasn't much further than the Crooked Billet at the end of the street I lived in. The pub was dark, dingy, mouldy, populated mostly by elderly alcoholics who had totally given up on the idea of ever doing anything useful again in their lives, and it reeked of death. It was exactly the right kind of pub for the frame of mind I was in.

One afternoon I got chatting to Mingus, a local blues musician who had been involved with Core Arts and Genesis P. Orridge's Coum Transmissions. After he introduced me to some of his friends another pub, known locally as the Wanker, came into the conversation, and I suggested that it had a reputation for easily available hard drugs. Mingus and his crew, who often drank at the Wanker, were incensed by this suggestion and insisted on inspecting my arms for non-existent track marks, thinking I looked the sort, and then banished me from their table. The following day Eddie Murray arrived at my flat to borrow the seven feet long Reclaim Bedlam syringe sculpted by Cat Monstersmith, to use for a live art piece he was scheduled to perform the next day. I told him about the argument at the Crooked Billet and he suggested that we should go there, watch the football and cause trouble, taking the syringe with us. As we sat with our pints and giant needle, we were challenged. *"What the fuck are you doing with that thing?"* a man I came to know as Alan Sarsfield demanded.

"We've got very big habits, mate!" Eddie shot back. Crooked Billet regulars warmed to me later, and I handwrote most of the first draft of this book in the place. Eddie never returned the syringe because, later that year, he attempted to hang himself with a rope dangling from outside his kitchen window in Ladbroke Grove. However, the rope snapped and it was the tarmac several floors below that killed him. Giving a speech at a wake held mostly for family members, I recalled the pub incident with the syringe, and it was obvious from his sisters' nervous looks that they'd thrown the prop into a skip during the sorting out his possessions. Eddie, a trained lawyer, had won a few thousand pounds a year previously from a housing association he'd been in dispute with, resolving to spend his windfall on 'wine, women and song'. And he spent the year doing just that, checking out when the money ran out.

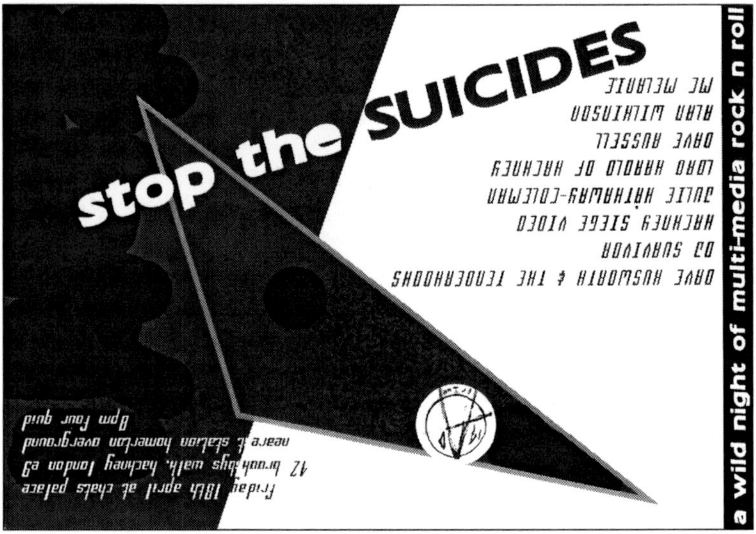
stop the SUICIDES
a wild night of multi-media rock n roll

Life wound down, and over the next few months Crooked Billet days were punctuated by the occasional show hosted by Mad Pride or Southwark Mind. Penny Shaughnessy, with nowhere to go after her husband's suicide, moved into my spare room and I also began spending time with Shirley Pearson after Gini and myself went our separate ways. A Southwark Mind leaving do was held for me at Camberwell Jazz Crypt in February, organised by Sarah Taylor, entirely without my advance knowledge. Ben and Esther had pretended to invite me and Gini out for a meal, and when we neared our supposed south bank destination in a taxi I was blindfolded, taken to the venue and led inside, where 150 friends awaited me, including several poets and musicians. Unwisely, people chose to put bottles of red wine in front of me and, overwhelmed and unworthy, I quickly lost the plot. Most of the show was recorded from the mixing desk, which was just as well because I couldn't remember much of it afterwards. Performers included Alan Tyler, Frank Bangay, Dave Russell, Ben Watson, Kelly Brown, Tony Palfrey, Julie Hathaway and Rick Henderson's band Arnie, and some of the show was released later that year on the live album *The Bad Boys of Mental Health: A Year in the Life of Mad Pride and Southwark Mind.* Apparently Hugh Mulhall helped get me home in a taxi after the event had finished.

There was an inquest for Pete attended by myself, Penny, Shirley and other people we didn't know. Inevitably, the jury re-

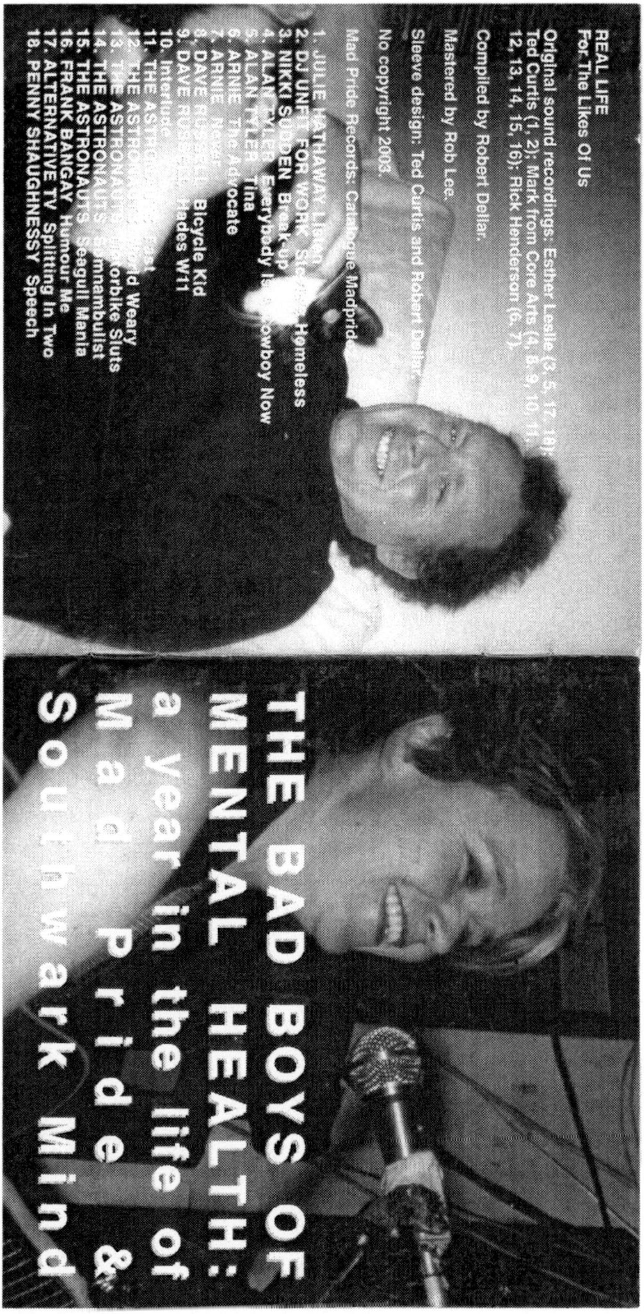

The Bad Boys of Mental Health: A Year int he Life of Mad Pride and Southwark Mind, front cover

turned the verdict that Pete had killed himself while the balance of his mind had been disturbed. Self-styled user activist Rosemary Moore, who claimed she had met Pete on one single occasion, turned up and treated the event as a fun day out, taking photographs of the coroner's court which she then gleefully published online as part of her web magazine *Mental*. She even managed to manoeuvre herself into the dock to give 'evidence', consisting of recitals of articles Pete and I had written for *Southwark Mind Newsletter*, in order to aggrandise herself. If Pete had been there he might have been amused; but we weren't.

The rest of the *Bad Boys* album was compiled from recordings of two further shows. Mad Pride held a 'Stop the Suicides' event at Chat's Palace on Good Friday 2003, headlined by Dave Kusworth and announcing a campaign which never went much further than the manufacture of hundreds of button badges and stickers. Remarkably, Dave was sober, having undergone a medically-assisted detox a few weeks previously. It was the first and only time I ever saw him sing and play guitar unintoxicated, and he seemed unusually nervous, although his heartbreaking, melodic rock songs went down well with the crowd, as did his unfeasibly skinny leather trousers. Phil Murphy, calling himself DJ Unfit For Work, performed his first show for seven years, singing over backing tapes of computer-generated pop and writhing about on the floor of the stage like the madman he was. Other acts included Julie Hathaway, Dave Russell, Tom who was Gini's new saxophonist boyfriend, and the elderly writer Sir Harold of Hackney. Sir Harold, whose real name was Ralph Levene, was a regular at Pumpkins and one-time associate of Samuel Beckett, Alexander Trocchi, James Joyce and Orson Welles, and his furiously bitter prose, given free rein in his late-period novel *The Mortician's Beauty Parlour* – which is about a necrophiliac prowling the streets of Tower Hamlets – was entirely suitable for the occasion.

Premiered at this event was Gini's new film, which concerned the longest siege ever held in Britain, in Graham Road in central Hackney a few weeks previously. A young, armed black gangster had held the filth at bay from a flat above a newsagent for over two weeks, his hostage only escaping when the hoodie finally fell asleep for a while. Where I lived in Hackney, exactly at the centre of the area referred to by tabloids as Murder Mile, somebody or other was shot once a week without fail, usually as a result of disputes between rival crack-dealing gangs. Ritually, the same stretch of Upper Clapton Road, near to the Lea Bridge roundabout, was cordoned off each week with yellow tape attached to poles by the old bill. After a few days the cordon would be removed, only to reappear after the next shooting: I don't know why they didn't just leave it there permanently to save time. So the siege didn't seem like a big deal locally, but it was a national media event. Even when the hostage escaped, police were reluctant to steam in, worried about the gangster's firepower. Armed with her video recorder, Gini interviewed the police, the staff at the nearby kebab shop who reported that their sales were down, the beggar who sat outside the adjacent branch of Woolworths every day and who suggested calling in the SAS, the gangster's friend who was caught trying to smuggle skunk to the gunman inside a takeaway KFC, and regulars at the Ship in Mare Street, the Sylvester Passage back entrance of which was closed off when all of this was going on. Drinking there during the siege made me imagine Derry during the troubles, watching cops in paramilitary gear pacing up and down the alleyway at the back with rifles trained on imaginary targets. The hoodie died eventually after he set fire to the flat. The cause of his death was never entirely clear: he may have been burnt alive, he may have died as the police claimed from a self-inflicted gunshot to the head, or he may have been shot dead by the police, who pulled the trigger a fair few times during the siege's tragic denouement. However, the hoodie didn't die in vain, because a short film came out of it which was shown at Chat's Palace on Good Friday 2003.

Following another show at Camberwell Jazz Crypt featuring the Arlenes and Alan Tyler to launch the paperback of Southwark Mind's manifesto, two tribute concerts took place for Pete, the first of them in May at the Foundry, the location of Mad Pride's first ever show. An intimate event for a hundred or so of Pete's close friends and work colleagues, who drank the bar dry, it featured musical performances by the usual suspects. Several people spoke from the stage, including Penny's teenage son Dan, who gave a particularly moving tribute to his stepdad. With the help of Penny Shaughnessy and Simon Holder, Gini had created yet another film, *Endless Love*, a celebration of Pete's life, and its first screening took place in the Foundry's basement art gallery against a wall beside a banner announcing someone's art exhibition called *No War but the Class War*. The film contained footage of Pete ranting on stage, being interviewed on TV shows about user-led mental health issues, and walking down Worthing High Street looking cool in his shades and Mad Pride t-shirt, Ceramic Hobs' 'Make Mine a Large One' blasting out in the background.

The next and more widely publicised show was at the Garage in Highbury on Summer Solstice night, again featuring the *Endless Love* video, trailed as a 'live video link-up from purgatory'. Several hundred people turned up to witness short sets by Alternative TV, Nikki Sudden, the Fish Brothers, Ceramic Hobs, Melanie Clifford, and a grunge band from up north. Melanie's set was especially moving, including as it did a song simply called 'Pete', during which Melanie scratched the word 'Pete' onto a pane of glass with a razor blade whilst screeching eerily, with her friend Rob adding atonal guitar accompaniment. Finally Penny Shaughnessy gave a moving speech, a recording of which was released on the *Bad Boys* album.

And that's a fraction of what happened, and what happened next really doesn't matter.

Death Disco

Some of my erstwhile colleagues attempted to keep Mad Pride ticking over but for me the buzz had gone, and worse, Mad Pride was starting to sell out by co-operating with clinicians such as Dr Rufus May and talking about putting the stockpile of weapons out of commission. It stood to reason that a splinter group had to be created, which I decided to call Continuity Mad Pride. To minimise the risk of the group being infiltrated by secret services, or diluted by those who wished to moderate all that we'd ever stood for, I resolved that the new group should consist only of myself.

It was around this time that I changed my appearance. Now that I didn't have to hold down a job, I no longer wore the suit and tie that had previously given me a veneer of respectability and instead took to dressing in punk rags like the kids I remembered from the Wapping Autonomy Centre, and I developed a mohican hairstyle like Wattie from the Exploited. I had commissioned a network of spies, at arm's length so that they weren't aware of who their actual handler was, to find out what some of the mental health professionals working in Hackney got up to behind the scenes, and so I had heard some of the rumours. But it took an uncanny sequence of events for me to properly piece it all together.

When I awoke in the morning twilight I was hungover, it was fucking freezing, and it took me a minute or so to work out where I was. And then it clicked. I'd spent the previous evening in the Jolly Butchers in Stoke Newington High Street, and I had only meant to hang around for a short while afterwards in the cemetery opposite the pub to pay homage to the great Salvation Army founder Sir William Booth who was buried there, but I must have nodded off. I checked my pockets. Blast! All my money had gone – every penny! Some cunt must have picked my pockets during the night! My head ached, and my body felt stiff from the cold and from having slept in an awkward position on top of Sir Bill's tomb. I was dying for a fag. I patted my pockets, checking once more. No fags! I looked at my watch to check the time. My watch had gone! The cunt must have taken that as well! At least the scoundrel hadn't taken my Mohican! I guessed from the twitter of the birds that it was roughly six in the morning. Far too early: what a fucking awful time to wake up!

I staggered towards the cemetery gates, walking past Jim MacDougall who appeared to be rubbing his cock against a gravestone. Fortunately he didn't notice me and I made it out onto the High Street, where I saw five middle-aged men in suits coming in my direction. As they drew closer I overheard their conversation.

"*I say, it was awfully decent of the pharmaceutical company to treat us to the free night's entertainment at the high-class Stamford Hill brothel, wouldn't you say, Tarquin?*" said one of the bastards with an accent dripping with privilege and education. "*I shall certainly be prescribing their new line of anti-psychotic medication to my patients, starting from today!*"

"*And I shall be following your good example, Oliver!*" said another cunt. "*The better the launch party, the finer the product, what?*"

I was suspicious of what they were saying but they looked rich, so I resolved to tap them for some dosh if I could. I reeled towards the quintet and begged. "*Here mate*" I enquired, "*You couldn't do us a favour, like, could you? I'm a bit short, like, I got thieved, and I can't fuckin' get home. Lend us a couple of quid for the bus fare, please kind sirs, and I'll pay you back the next time I see you.*"

"*Most certainly not, young man*" the shrink replied, "*learn to stand on your own two feet!*" The other four laughed at their colleague's amusing joke.

"*Got a spare fag, then?*" I asked.

"*We don't smoke, I'm sure!*"

"What about you, then?" I said turning to another one. *"You look like you've got a few bob. It won't hurt you, like, helping out another human being for a change. Got two quid?"*

"Push off, you lout!" the toff replied, pushing me gently out of the way. I'd worked it out. He'd had a hard night shagging his pick of the top Stamford Hill tarts courtesy of the manufacturers of the latest psychiatric wonder drug. After this ordeal, he probably figured he was at least entitled to a hassle-free walk to the hospital so that he could grab a couple of hours' kip behind his desk before starting work. But I didn't like being pushed and I was in a very bad mood. Snarling, I clenched my fist into a tight ball and lashed out viciously at the off-duty psychiatrist, smacking him in the mouth. The bastard keeled over backwards spitting blood: he'd lost four of his teeth!

Unwisely one of his colleagues, who looked a bit like the eminent Bevan ward consultant Dr Lucey, decided to remonstrate. *"Now, young man, you may very well have had a deprived childhood, and you may indeed be suffering from diminished responsibility! But think about this: what does violence ever achieve?"* His romantic exploits over the past few hours had been spiced with a few too many lines of cocaine.

It was strange how these doctors insisted on referring to me as a young man when some of them were probably a fair few years younger than me, though they were already fat and going bald. Taking this as patronising, I stiffened, tense. Then quick as a flash I grabbed hold of the Lucey lookalike's combed-over hair, used it to pull the shrink's head down, and jabbed my steel toe-capped boot up hard and sharp into his face, shattering the cunt's expensive dental work which had been designed to give him a Donny Osmond smile, whilst simultaneously flattening the bastard's nose. The other doctors gasped and whimpered in sympathy with their assailed co-worker.

By chance a siren's wail approached up the high street, from the direction of the nearby filth station. I knew what that meant: time to run for it!

As I shot up Northwold Road, the shrinks flagged down the Black Maria and pointed the cops towards me. I reached Rectory Road; the siren's decibel count increased. I ran faster, drawing on hidden reserves of energy, my head pounding, until the van drew up alongside me and the coppers flew out. I kept running, more in defiance now than hope; a pig dive-bombed me with a rugby tackle. I struggled: I wasn't going to let the scumbag take me alive. I turned, twisted, and kicked out from a carefully contrived angle, managing to catch the cop sharply in the groin and ensuring that the bastard's wedding tackle would be out of commission for the next few months. As the cop doubled up clutching his bollocks in unbearable agony, the other pigs jumped on top of me and collectively dragged me down to the pavement. The last thing I remembered after I regained consciousness was the feel of the boots raining hard and fast into my head, chest, stomach, groin, everywhere really; those sickening sensations of pain and helplessness before I blacked out.

When I awoke I didn't know where the fuck I was. It was the second time in succession that I'd woken up with that kind of disorientated feeling. Before, I'd felt terrible because of a hangover. This time however, an entirely new sensation had taken hold: I was bombed out, and I felt like a fucking zombie. I couldn't concentrate at all. My vision was blurred and inanimate objects seemed to sway in front of me. I was shaking a little and rocking in a chair: it was well strange, and wherever it was that I was seemed haunted, as if tormented ghosts were lurking quietly in the background. My body was aching and sore from my kicking at the hands of the old bill, especially my ribs, and the zombie feeling felt akin to nothing previously familiar. Where was I?

I was in a small hall. Through the blur I could discern several other human figures. Most of them were crashed out in chairs, or else littered in ungainly positions across the floor or on cushions. They looked as if someone had dropped them there from the ceiling like lifeless rag dolls, so random were the slumbering shapes they assumed. Watching over them were bouncer characters who looked as hard as nails, ready and willing to pounce at the least provocation. I looked out of the window: I was on the third floor of an old building. Too fragile to risk antagonising the bouncers, too scared to even try to scrounge a fag, I resolved to keep a low profile while I tried to work out just what the fuck was going on.

I was left alone for a while until one of the bouncers approached. *"It's time for you to meet the doctor!"* he announced, making me stand up and locking my arms behind my back in a vicelike custodial grip. *"You'll like the doctor! Now, let's move, punk!"*

I had trouble making my muscles move. With great effort I marched at the security man's pace. My wrists ached and I could

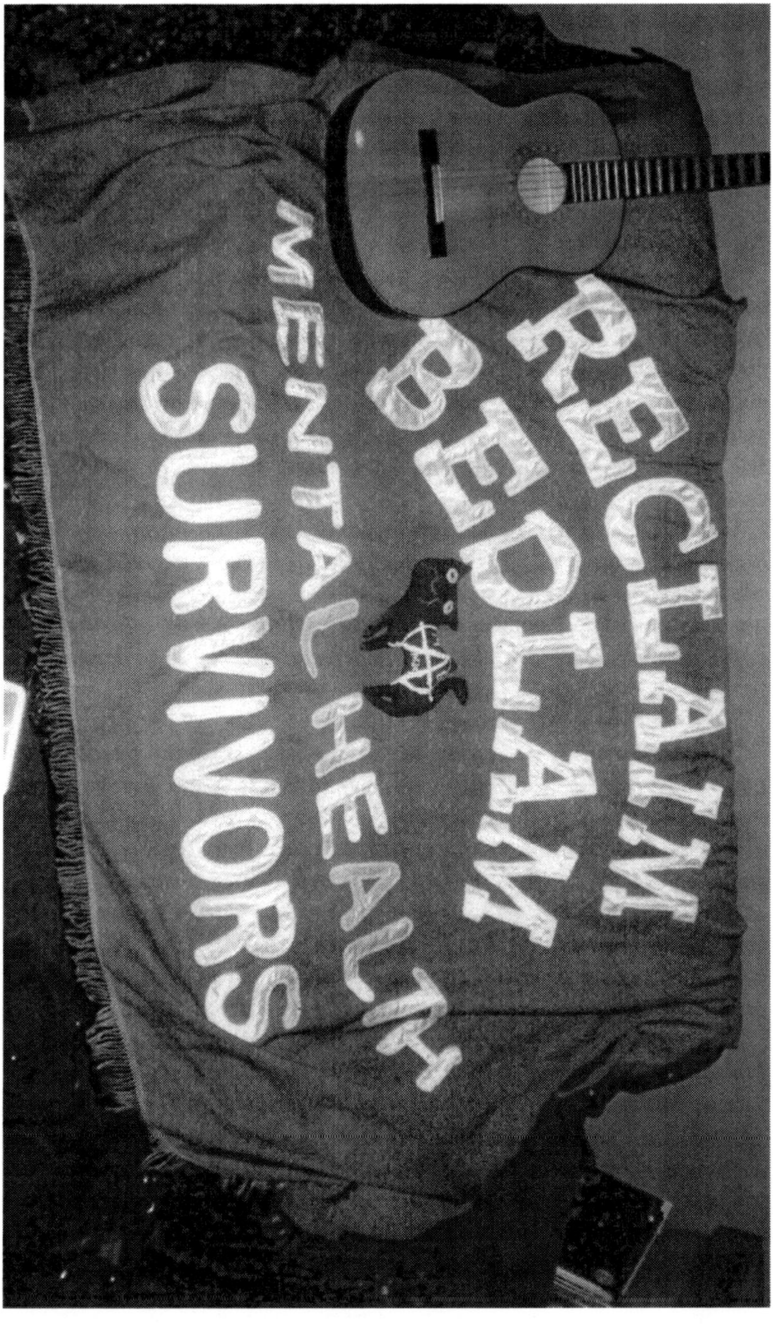
RECLAIM
BEDLAM
MENTAL HEALTH
SURVIVORS

tell that I'd been in handcuffs, but this didn't appear to be a police station. It seemed more like PICU, infamously the hardest and most violent ward in the Hackney hospital prior to its closure in 1994. And then the realisation struck me: IT WAS PICU! Either I'd been transported back in time, or the dreaded lock-up had secretly been reopened. I was frog-marched to the shrink's office, anger welling up deep within my soul. I wasn't a fucking loony!

When I entered the office I had another shock: the doctor was one of the cunts who'd sent the cops after me! Unfortunately he wasn't one of those I'd beaten up; it would have cheered me a little to see some of the fruits of my labour. I strained against the wrist-lock: I wanted to rectify my omission and smash the fuck out of this doctor as well, but the bouncer's grip was firm and I felt strangely weak. Resigned, I sat down when commanded to do so.

"*Good morning Mr Dellar*" the shrink said superciliously while looking at his notes. "*We've met before, haven't we?*" I could see the wicked irony in his eyes when he looked up and added: "*I say, it was jolly good luck that you met my good self and my colleagues yesterday in Stoke Newington, otherwise your mental illness might never have received the treatment it so clearly requires!*"

"*Fuck you, you cunt*" I hissed.

"*Fortunately, when we discovered that you had been intercepted by the constabulary, we managed to persuade them that it was in your own best interests for you to be diverted here and not to the cells. It would appear that you had a minor altercation with the police, but they were gracious enough to decline to press charges.*" The evil doctor smirked, a grin of pure malevolent hatred. He was pleased that I was covered in bruises and dried blood and had several broken ribs. And if he had anything to do with it, my corporal punishment at the hands of the old bill would only be the start of my treatment!

"*During your stay at Hackney psychiatric hospital, we're going to try you out on a variety of psychotropic medications*" he explained, introducing himself as Dr Tarquin Forbes-Windsor. "*We're starting you off with Haloperidol, because that's a particularly nasty, sorry, slip of the tongue, effective medicine. We gave you a shot earlier while you were still unconscious. If you're still presenting psychotic symptoms after a few days, we'll try some Depixol on top. Because your condition is severe and enduring, we'll have to give you the maximum doses of course.*" Forbes-

Windsor suddenly collapsed into wild, spontaneous cackling. What a hoot! It was just so funny! He couldn't stop laughing!

"I'm gonna fucking kill you" I said, calm, serious and cold, staring straight into the doctor's eyes. It was a promise, not a threat, and the shrink belted up: it wasn't so funny anymore. I spat at him hatefully, leaving an extended strand of glutinous green gob dangling from his nose as the bouncer led me out of the room and towards the drugs cabinet. I was still stiff and sore from my beating and spaced out from the injection I'd had already, and I was fucked if I was letting the cunts give me another jab.

While the bouncer was fiddling with his syringe, loading the barrel with Haloperidol ready to squirt into my arse, I glimpsed the chance I was looking for. Another bouncer was unlocking the PICU door to let a cleaner in. As soon as it was open I shot towards it like a bullet from a pistol, simultaneously picking up a chair and smashing it brutally into the second bouncer's face so hard that the chair broke apart into splinters! The keys swung from the keyhole as the bouncer fell screaming to the floor, sorry for himself, holding his head in his hands, failing to stem the flow of blood as it spurted like a geyser from his horrific facial injuries.

For good measure, I booted the bastard in the stomach while he was down. Then, before anyone could react, I removed the keys, leapt through the door, pushed the cleaner aside, slammed the door, locked it from outside and darted off. My injuries hurt like fuck: it was a miracle that I could fucking move! But I would allow neither the pain nor the anti-psychotic stupor to spoil my chances as I raced down the stairs. I hadn't even reached the ground floor when the alarms went off: piercing, high-pitched wails, as loud and shrill as I remembered them from the fireworks party held on the hospital site nine years earlier. Pounding feet were barely audible from ahead compared to this aural assault as I hurtled towards the exit, but I knew that security staff were rushing to prevent my departure. Desperately, I tried a nearby door and, finding it unlocked, I jumped inside to hide.

I found myself in a room full of people drinking cans of Tennents Super, passing round spliffs, and dancing to roots reggae as it blasted from a cassette recorder. Posters everywhere bore slogans like 'Fuck the mental health system', 'Psychiatry? No thanks' and 'The only good shrink is a dead shrink', echoing my sentiments exactly.

"This is the hospital advocacy office", said a friendly woman holding a paintbrush and standing by a canvas, making a portrait of a nude character sitting on a chair in front of her. *"What can we do you for?"* She had to shout, because the alarm was so noisy.

"I've just done a bunk from the wards upstairs and the cunts are after me, know what I mean?" I said.

"Don't worry" said the artist, getting some keys out and using one of them to unlock a door. *"If you hide in this cupboard, we might let you out when everything's calmed down."* She seemed unfazed, as if escapees covered in blood and bruises were part and parcel of her usual work routine. I had nothing to lose, so I hopped in. The door shut behind me and a key turned, locking me inside.

Moments later there was a knock on the advocacy door followed by a voice: stern, official and authoritative, making itself heard above the din. *"We're looking for a particularly dangerous patient who's just escaped from upstairs,"* it said. *"He has kind of a mohican hairstyle. Any of you lot seen him?"*

"No, he's not here, but if we find him, we'll let you know."

"Nice one" said the guard, leaving, and after a while the sirens stopped. I sat in the cupboard thinking about how Falklands Andy must have felt way back then in Camden Road, as I began to recover my strength and consider my strategy. I'd had a tough and painful time and I was desperate for a fag. I ached all over thanks to the police, and my head still felt confused courtesy of the haloperidol, but nevertheless I felt murderously angry. Somebody was going to have to pay for this, I thought as the advocate let me out of the cupboard.

Meanwhile the ward round was held in a small room upstairs in PICU, and Tarquin Forbes-Windsor sat in the largest chair, as befitted his position of authority. The pill-pusher had established himself as one of the top consultant psychiatrists in East London, and in the region of a hundred grand a year, his job was a profitable one – without even taking into account the perks that frequently came his way in the form of the tasty female patients and female doctors who passed through. He looked around the room proudly. It was his. Nobody could challenge his control. He was the high priest of PICU, performing ceremonies, rites, initiations, exorcisms: his every word a shining nugget of sacred wisdom. He was surrounded by junior shrinks on placement at the hospital, learning their trade. Even by the normal standards, Forbes-Windsor seemed to reflect, this lot looked like a sorry shower. The three remaining boys were all spotty, chinless inadequates in grey suits, with trousers too short for them which revealed navy blue socks and polished brown shoes. They were depleted in number because the consultant had just sent the fourth one home for not wearing a tie. I could see all of this because there was a bank of TV screens in the advocacy office showing live footage of the various parts of the hospital where the advocates had secretly installed closed circuit TV cameras. Additionally, hidden microphones were somehow wired up to the beat box, every word upstairs audible now that the reggae had been switched off. Andy Martin, who had just appeared in the office in the course of doing his Hackney Patients Council rounds, filled me in on all of the details and gave me some tobacco.

The two female junior doctors, one big, the other small, wore smart dresses and nondescript haircuts: they didn't look anything special but Forbes-Windsor wasn't too fussy, he'd still shagged the bigger of the two earlier that morning. Despite the weak impression the juniors made, the boss contented himself with an intuition generated by his many years' experience telling him that one day, they'd all grow up to be adult psychiatrists just like him.

Even though he was pissed off that I'd escaped, the doctor liked his job, which was equally divided between dishing out medication and shagging. The junior he'd supervised before the ward round had known full well that keeping her seniors happy was the best way of ensuring a smooth transition into a medical career, and despite being deficient on the looks front, Forbes-Windsor knew he was onto a good thing. But he wasn't satisfied with just the one romantic escapade. It was barely midday, leaving plenty of time ahead for further conquests. Now he was meeting his other new patients one by one for the first time, diagnosing their complaints and prescribing the appropriate gear to subdue them as the baby shrinks watched. He worked with the calm and confident manner of a true professional, but inside he was concentrating less on the matter in hand than on which patient would follow the young doctor he'd shagged already onto his couch. After seeing the first few new faces he reflected that the quality wasn't up to much. If nothing better came along, he'd probably knock off for the day after shagging the smaller of the two female juniors.

Forbes-Windsor had a tried and tested method of getting what he wanted from the PICU girls. He'd give them a large injection and a selection of weird pills and potions which knocked them out to the extent that they barely noticed him shagging them in his office. And if their largactyl-addled brains showed any sign of recalling the doctor's exploits later, he'd simply give them a few shots of electro-convulsive therapy, which would erase all traces of recent memory. Even this sometimes failed, but luckily it was always the patient's word against his, and nobody would ever take the word of someone locked up because they were insane against that of a top psychiatrist. The doctor got a satisfactory result every time. And although his colleagues had one or twice in the past been caught out over similar behaviour, he felt secure in the knowledge that such instances were always hushed up and forgotten by the medical establishment, keeping the offenders safely in their jobs. This was only fair, he reflected. Consultant psychiatrists deserved the privilege, warranted by the depth of their expertise, of taking their pick of the women on the wards.

The ward round continued. The shrink was treating it as a beauty parade, awarding the females in the procession marks out of ten in his head as they passed. They all received low marks until an attractive Chinese patient who couldn't speak a word of English was carted in. The doctor awarded her eight marks. Given the state of the competition, she'd won by a mile: she was this week's Miss PICU!

He went through the motions of giving her a decent assessment. He looked her up and down a bit, checking for delusions. Stared her out, seeing if he could spot any grandiose thoughts. Walked over and prodded her a few times to check out her response. Then he sat back in his seat, wrote out her medication chart for the week, and turned to the nurse sitting next to him. "*It looks like a bad case of schizo-affective disorder to me!*" he explained. "*We'll need to give her an extra-special, high dose of Olanzipine and various other medicines that I've prescribed in order to get her safely on the road to recovery. When the tablets and injections have had time to work, she'll be as right as rain! Now, I'll need to give this patient a special examination later on, so you should bring her to my office at two o'clock.*"

The nurse nodded. He had his suspicions but knew that if he voiced them he'd be sacked. He wasn't too bothered in any case: nurses had their own methods of obtaining favours from their patients. People had been known to die in hospitals from overdoses of psychiatric drugs, I thought to myself, often on their way to or from dubious special examinations with consultants such as the one being arranged with the Chinese chick. The ODs were always covered up, explained away in coroners' reports as being everyday heart attacks. People dropped dead all the time from the effects of their medication. Nobody gave a fuck. Mental patients had limited rights at the best of times, and once they wound up on PICU – which didn't officially exist, having been closed down nine years earlier in 1994 – every aspect of their lives was under the control of the nurses and, especially, the doctors. Each death became nothing more than another statistic, manoeuvred into a misleading column.

The ward round ended and Forbes-Windsor strode happily back to his office elsewhere in the building. The Chinese girl looked well fit, and her lack of mastery of the English tongue would be an extra safeguard against detection. If things worked out for them on the couch as well as he hoped, he mused, it might even be worth extending her section.

On his way to his office he passed Dr Oliver Coyde, who was no relation to the similarly surnamed erstwhile boss of the Interim Secure Unit, but who nevertheless was escorting an attractive and heavily-tranquilised female patient back to her unit after a special examination; the two doctors winked at each other conspiratorially, mindful of the rewards that went with their medical knowledge. A few yards later Forbes-Windsor bumped into the smaller of the two women juniors: the one he hadn't shagged yet. The baby shrink was eager to further her career and knew that she'd need a good reference from the consultant. She was only too pleased to accept his suggestion that she should accompany him to his office for an extracurricular supervision session. The new Chinese patient was the top item on the doctor's menu, but there was time for everyone: he had all afternoon.

As he drew the blinds and supervised the junior to strip, he thought about the power he had over his staff, his patients, over the whole hospital, a hospital which didn't even exist and which therefore barely had to be accounted for. He reflected that his mastery was no more than a man of his eminent professional status deserved. His power generated his libido. The junior took her orders from the learned professional who earned a six figure sum annually, and spread herself passively over the top of the desk. Forbes-Windsor removed his own clothes except for his lucky public school tie, then he climbed on top of the prostrate trainee and gave her the benefit of his specialist clinical expertise. He took his time over the clinical assessment, demonstrating carefully his superior medical wisdom. The key to a successful transaction between a doctor and his patient was the skill with which the superior made his examination, revealing the site of his subject's complaint in the harsh, all-seeing glare of the clinical gaze. Watching it on TV, Andy Martin got his cock out from his track suit trousers and had a wank. As soon as the doctor felt that his analysis was complete and that he had a thorough understanding of his patient's symptoms, it was time for him to make his diagnosis and issue forth his prescription.

Satisfied that his medication had worked and puffing and panting a little from the exertion, he dismounted and ordered the junior to get her clothes back on and leave, adding that she had a fine future as a doctor ahead of her. It had been a thoroughly professional liaison.

Andy explained to me that the local mental health trust had reopened PICU clandestinely as a pilot scheme, so that they could deal with difficult to manage patients without scrutiny, and without having to adhere to all of the safeguards contained in the 1983 mental health act. There was a very experimental aspect to the illicit ward, and its results were being carefully monitored by her majesty's Department of Health which was thinking about possibly opening similar secret hospital wards elsewhere. The installation of an advocacy service on the site was a part of the experiment, as was the token involvement of Hackney Patients Council. Andy didn't really do anything; he just dropped in from time to time to keep up appearances, and the trust had given him a pay rise in exchange for him keeping quiet.

I had a score to settle. Forbes-Windsor, still in full view on a TV screen in the advocacy room, was alone in his own office with the blinds drawn, and he was going to be made to pay for the collective sins of his profession. He was swigging from a bottle of vodka contentedly, waiting for the nurse to deliver his afternoon treat. The small junior doctor had gone and the next girl wasn't due for an hour, so he had plenty of time to put his clothes back on. He'd locked himself in to avoid interruption, and was pleased just to relax and enjoy the uninhibited comfort of his own nakedness. He took another hit of vodka, lit a cigar and looked forward to the promising afternoon's work ahead.

Following Andy's directions, and having borrowed some items which I thought I might need from the advocacy stationery cupboard, I made it to Forbes-Windsor's office unchallenged in no time. Knowing that the door was locked, I raised my right foot into the air, slowly, until it was in a kicking position. I kept myself balanced in that poise for a moment, concentrating, and then with a sudden, great rush of energy surging from every part of my body straight into my right leg, I lashed out, booting the door off its hinges in one go. As it crashed to the ground I beheld the fat, almost bald bastard smoking a cigar, drinking vodka and wearing not a stitch save for his lucky public school tie which he never removed under any circumstances.

I'd taken the doctor by surprise. I whipped out a stanley knife and pressed it against my victim's throat. "*One move, one sound out of you, and you're dead, cunt. Got it?*" I hissed. I wasn't joking.

Now holding my blade menacingly between my teeth, my eyes wild, I bound my patient's wrists and ankles with a ball of string. Forbes-Windsor's clothes were on top of a filing cabinet, neatly folded. I got the underpants and stuffed them into the shrink's mouth before wrapping the socks tightly round his head, ensuring that he could neither see nor scream. Then I tied the doctor to his desk with a length of rope. I lit a fag; sucked hard on it, and then I stubbed it out on his chest, making him wriggle mutely like a severed segment of a giant pink earthworm. I swigged from the vodka thirstily as I searched the office with a keen sense of purpose. Inside the filing cabinet I found a drawer containing just what I needed: a party-sized selection of syringes, pills, and bottles of anti-psychotic solutions.

After putting on a pair of rubber gloves I got two spoons and crushed a variety of tablets into a fine powder. Then I took a bottle of clozapine, unscrewed the cap, poured the powder in, replaced the cap, and shook it until the particles had dissolved. Pleased with the blend, I loaded the barrel of a syringe with the heavily tranquilising syrup.

"*The trouble with you psychiatrists*" I told him, "*is that you force people to have all these pills and injections all the time, without having personally experienced their efficacy. Know what I mean? You'll be a much better doctor once this omission has been rectified!*" The shrink struggled a little as he felt the contents of the syringe empty into his mainline, but the knots I'd tied held firm. I cackled in a friendly kind of way. "*This will make you feel better, mate*" I told him as I squeezed the juice into Forbes-Windsor's bloodstream. *"Sitting around in an office wearing nothing but a tie is classified as a symptom of schizophrenia in the manual!"*

The doctor made a last vain attempt to free himself of his bondage before the shot took effect, depriving him of the ability to move. I lit another fag and, for the hell of it, began identifying with the psychiatrist's role, and I took the shrink's resistance to taking his medication as evidence of his lack of insight into the nature of his mental illness. Obviously he'd need further treatment before his condition stabilised. I mixed another cocktail and gave the shrink a second injection. When the second dose kicked in the doctor found that he was struggling to maintain consciousness. His entire existence was being nullified by the pharmaceutical agents of social control. Suddenly, he felt a series of involuntary muscular spasms overwhelm his bulk and he jolted violently as the overdose played havoc with his neural transmission system. He was in the throes of a major psychiatrically-induced fit!

I'd decided on this course of action because I'd been reminded of the theoretical difficulties I had with the discipline of psychiatry, which saw distress and mad behaviour as an illness caused by genetic and biochemical factors, rather than as a legitimate response to a sad world in which 'sane' responses had proved themselves inadequate. Psychiatrists were hand in glove with the large multinational pharmaceutical companies, and together they were forever looking for new markets onto which to push their products, typically against the wishes of the punters taking them. It was all about big business, money, and power, as a result of which it sometimes felt as if patients were dropping like flies, falling victim to the debilitating side effects of their medication. Mind doctors had been committing genocide, waging a one-sided war on their clientele for years. But this war was one-sided no longer: doctors would be held accountable, and I was judge, jury and executioner.

"One of the problems with this medicine, right, is that it's a bit fucking ropey, know what I mean?" Troubled by the severity of Forbes-Windsor's fit, I crushed a quantity of procyclidine pills into dust and mixed them with liquid largactyl. *"To alleviate the nasty side effects, we'll have to give you some more medication, to act as an antidote to the enormous dose of drugs you've already had. Get my drift? Now,*

hold your breath, mate, and count to ten." I loaded the hypodermic once again and shot the contents into the doctor's arm.

He was still twitching spasmodically and making the occasional funny noise, which I took to be a sign of residual mental illness requiring one last top up of medication. I'd polished off most of the vodka and, having searched the doctor's pockets for his wallet, I knew I'd be sorted for further alcohol for a few days should I so wish and if I could reach an off licence. I poured some more neuroleptic solutions and crushed tablets into the last of the vodka, not even bothering to check the brand names, screwed the top back on and shook the bottle until the serum went fizzy. Then, after extracting a funnel from the filing cabinet, I removed the socks and underpants from the doctor's face, stuck the funnel into the shrink's mouth, and carefully, making sure that none of it was spilt, I decanted the anti-psychotic vodka into his throat. By the time it had all gone down, the nude consultant had stopped twitching and wasn't even presenting any observable symptoms. He'd been given a chemical lobotomy!

Satisfied that I'd done my bit for medical science by making an example of the overweight nymphomaniac, I cleared up the mess I'd made in the office. My argument was with psychiatrists, the police force and people like that, and I had no desire to create extra work for the hospital cleaning staff, who were underpaid and had enough to do already. Leaving my patient propped up naked against the filing cabinet, I left the office and wandered unchallenged back to the advocacy office, where I was given a standing ovation by the advocates who had been watching the whole episode on their CCTV screens. When the nurse visited the doctor a little later to deliver the desirable Chinese chick, rigor mortis had already started to set in. Unfortunately, the doctor had passed away.

The advocates took me to the entrance of a secret tunnel which led from the hospital to the Kingsmead Estate, and I walked home from there. After a few weeks I'd entirely recovered from my injuries, and the medication had worn off, although for a time I was nervous that the police or secret services might come and take me away. But for some reason they never bothered to do so, and I remain to this day a free man.

This Perfect Day

During the Paris uprisings of May 1968, interesting items of graffiti appeared on walls in reclaimed spaces, the most notorious sharing the slogan 'Beneath the paving stones, the beach'. Such words may or may not have been inspired by Guy Debord's Situationists. I wasn't there, and would only have been three at the time. But I gather there was another slogan, which simply said: 'Quick'. In French.

What apparently this meant was that the insurrection taking place at the time was itself the experience of freedom, and it was no guarantee of any future emancipation. Most people involved must have been aware that the French state, with all its resources and its army and police force, would effortlessly recapture the sectors of Paris briefly reoccupied by those of oppositional outlook. Only briefly would the protesters be able to take control of the streets, find the beach beneath the pavement if they felt so inclined, and breathe the ephemeral air of what must have felt, for a few moments, like freedom.

In retrospect it's easy to say that we should make the most of it while it lasts. At the time it's all too easy just to miss it, not truly realising or experiencing what happens in the moment. This is tragic, because nearly all glimpses of emancipation turn out to be merely momentary, and their preciousness can so easily be lost in a fog of planning and rationalisation. This does not, however, mean that these glimpses are illusions.

Conversely, the trouble with living through such events in the moment is that very little in the future ever seems quite so good, and what follows may seem something of a let down. I wasn't around in May 1968. I even missed the initial, authentic flourish of punk by being born three years too late. But my friends who were there during punk's early stages realise, looking back, that they were in on something special that can never be truly recreated, and a sad thing for some is that they weren't even aware of how special it was at the time. Maybe they thought that life could always be like that.

Two typical tendencies exist of people who have lived through such experiences. The first group enjoys nostalgia and dwelling in the past: not trying to recreate the intensity, but instead trying to find ways of remembering and celebrating it. The other involves romanticising that intensity, trying to find ways to simulate it, and perhaps looking for new situations where lessons learnt can be put to good use to create new, once again brief windows of freedom. Once that impulse is in your mind, it is hard to ever let it go.

This can't hold true for all of us. Some of the characters in this book have settled down with their mortgages and their kids, as they have every right to do, and are frightened of anything that reminds them of their wilder pasts or indeed, anything that takes them out of their security zones. Those people who have conformed have not always been the people who I would have anticipated doing so. Some of these people have not only opted for comfortable lives, but also reneged on their previous progressive political and social beliefs. These days, such people avoid me like the plague.

I've lived through a few all too brief approximations of emancipation, not always at the time having the confidence or presence of mind to realise what was happening. The anarchist centres in Wapping and Westbourne Park in the early 1980s, looking back on it, were special places where anything could and did happen, where I was surrounded by other kids who felt as alienated and outside of it all as I did – though, sadly, most of us felt so alienated that we didn't even realise that we all felt the same way, and we mostly failed to communicate with each other.

I've participated in several riots that I liked, and I can't wait for the next one.

Hackney Anarchy Week gave me some kind of a sensation of freedom, unwell though I was. It was a co-ordinated series of autonomous actions completely against the grain, and a few of us lived through it and got away with it, though unhappily I wasn't in a fit state to have experienced it with the sense of presence with which I would have liked to have done.

And most importantly for me, my work in the murky world of mental health helped lead to some precious times, including some of the outrageous stunts associated with City and Hackney Mind's advocacy service and later with Southwark Mind, and in particular, the stuff myself and a few others got up to calling ourselves Mad Pride. For such a short time, we really thought we could change the world. We were wrong, of course. Mad Pride was just a group of us who briefly made a lot of noise that made us sound bigger than we really were. We created a gratuitously intense time for ourselves, which was also lived vicariously by a few other people, and we paid the price.

After such experiences, everything else is tame. But, older and more tired as we become, some of us will always be keeping an eye open for the next opportunity: the appearance of something which at least feels, just for a second, like freedom; which imparts the visceral as well as cerebral sensations that we are truly alive, sensations that will remain with us in our memories and yearnings.

For some of us, the trust that this can still happen, if we truly want it to, is what makes it worth staying alive. Creating the brief flashes of what may as well be authentic and unmediated experience is the best that some of us can ever hope to achieve, because we are the people our parents warned us against.

Derelicts: Thought Worms From the Wreckage

Esther Leslie

ISBN: 978-0-9568176-9-3
Published: Mar 2014, 254pp

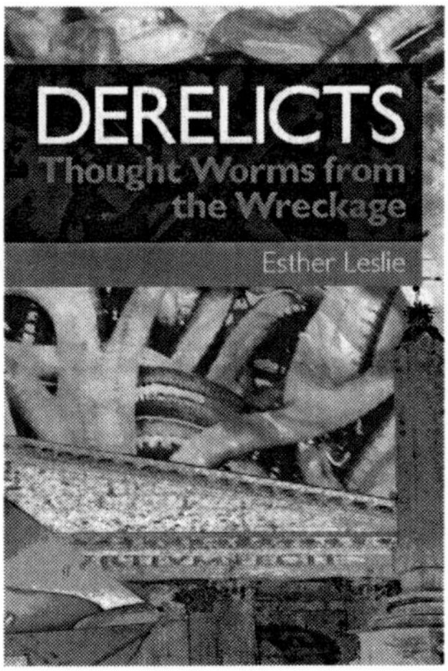

Philosophy and art with the imagination to actually change the world: this is the unfinished dream of history and the heart of the revolutionary modernism of the early 20th century, which globalised war and exploitation managed indefinitely to defer. Esther Leslie reopens the cold case on filmmakers, artists, thinkers and other animals, exiled or otherwise Disneyfied, and finds still-warm fertile ground for a wild future as yet unfulfilled. From ideal homes with traces erased to utopian rivers drawn back to their source, the alienated subject of history discerns its rightful place in the present tense, with no room for buts or half-measures. The derelicts of history find new life beyond commodified thought: would that the same could be said for all their readers.

Michael Tencer

Cosmic Orgasm: The Music of Iancu Dumitrescu

Andy Wilson (ed)

ISBN: 978-0-9568176-5-5
Published: May 2013, 406pp

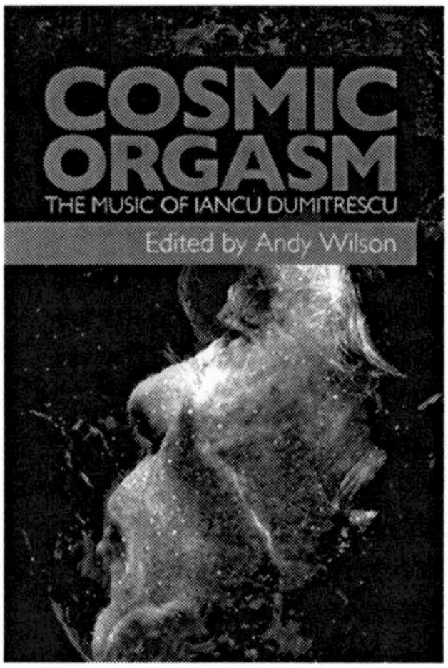

"As a creator of radical music that breaks convention, riding on the edge of the classical avant garde onto realms more closely associated with the likes of Nurse With Wound or The Hafler Trio, Iancu Dumitrescu has the talent to lure you in, mystify and startle with unnerving ferocity.

Alan Freeman

"Iancu Dumitrescu stands at the cutting edge of the whole range of new tendencies, representing a musical avant garde uncorrupted by compromise—in which the taste for invention merges with intellectual speculation in the philosophical sense of the word. As the outstanding figure in Romanian composed music, Iancu Dumitrescu developed from the 1970's the concept of acousmatic—a pre-Socratic term that refers to the art of concealing the sound source to render a message more mysterious "

George Astalos

"Of all living composers, Dumitrescu is the one who has most exploded sound. Dumitrescu's work is a negation, from the depths, of everything in contemporary music symptomatic of distraction, of banalisation, and of a radical loss of purpose. His music is not a new convolution in the knot of modern music, but an unravelling of the curse."

Tim Hodgkinson

Azmud

Ken Fox

ISBN: 978-0-9568176-4-8
Published: Mar 2013, 270pp

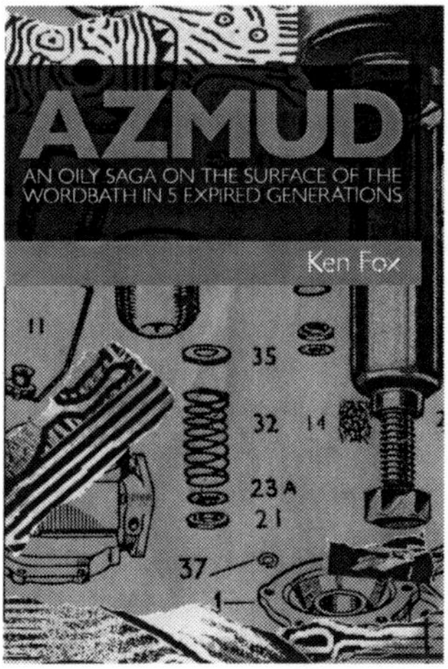

Drifting in & out of sense as in an interrupted dream, Azmud is a novel contribution to literary art as political allegory. In each of its five sections – 'expired generations' – it attempts to retell the tale of the human psyche, the damage it has undergone under capitalism, in the form of a wandering work tribe searching for value in the spectacular flow of mass communication, on behalf of various severe 'generals' who demand a quota of abstract accumulation. But each of Azmud's industrial adventures in turn become allegories for the act of the text's own creation. But what happens in Azmud? Under orders, a human herd wanders thru the dense miasma of mass communication, hunting for precious ox-ore to stash in their air-ark or fuel their ancient steam engine. A vagrant crew invades the broken dreams of a drowsy industrial tycoon, stealing baskets full of his precious sleep. A homeless hoard combs thru post-industrial litter, searching for burnable rubble. A fake engineer captures a team of lost work-horses & four mammoth protozoans to help boost the energy yield of his toxic currents. A cargo ship collects a crew of stranded industrial outcasts with their precious ark full of ore & its tyrannical captain subjects them to relentless injections & many unwanted adventures.

Association of Musical Marxists

More Years for the Locust

Jim Higgins

ISBN: 978-0-9568176-3-1
Published: Jun 2012, 330pp

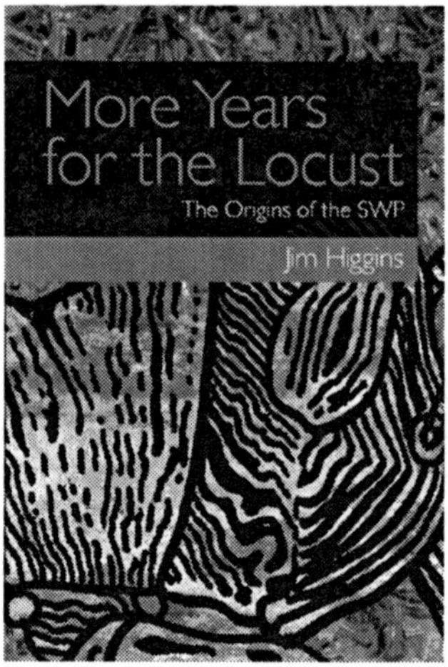

"There is a human scale to the story so often missing in the more staid accounts of the left and its history which often create an artificial barrier between readers and the activists being written about, who were after all, people much like them. This dimension of the book which, to put it bluntly, makes it such a good laugh, also provides a great store of what Aristotle would have called practical wisdom. The laughter and the nous are here very closely related and impossible to summarise, they must be read...

The trouble with Higgins is ultimately our own trouble. The reward for recognising this is to be able to rehabilitate and nourish a part of ourselves. The IS tradition is broader than the latest line or missive from the latest CC. This may seem a problem to some but it ought to be seen as a great resource. Revolutionaries too have traditions. Perhaps we are now in a position to learn from Higgins even if we were sadly a bit too stupid to do so before."

John Game, *Foreword*

Blake in Cambridge

Ben Watson

ISBN: 978-0-9568176-8-6
Published: Apr 2012, 168pp

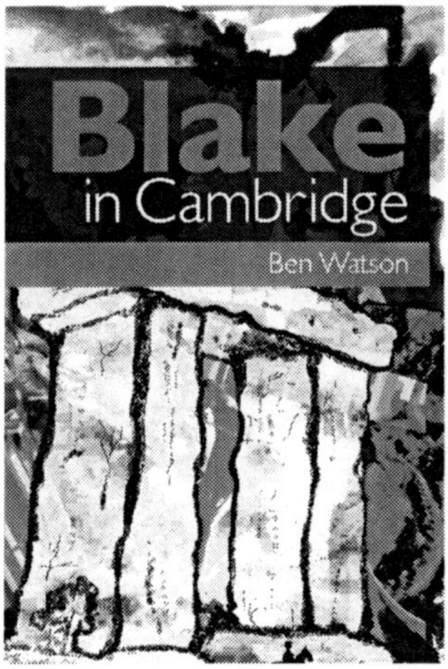

Blake in Cambridge was written after reading William Blake's visionary epic *Milton* during extended bouts of childcare in Coram's Fields in the summer of 2010. *Blake in Cambridge* is the Marxist critique of Eng. Lit. Christopher Caudwell was meant to write, but screwed up due to a CPGB sociology which denies literature the chance to answer back. In Marx's polemic, the jokes of *Tristram Shandy* and *Don Quixote* became weapons in class struggle. This, argues Watson, is how Blake can and should be used.

The **Association of Musical Marxists** says: A revolutionary party would not be paranoid about its members' proclivities. It would not try, like the Lindsey German-era SWP, to insulate members from avant garde extremes and bathe them, infant Cleopatras, in a dilute milk of inoffensive, politically-correct culture – soggy crumbs from the bosses' table. We need to pierce the veil of moralism and fear which protects the bourgeois racket. Blake for the masses! Start here...

1839: The Chartist Insurrection

Dave Black and Chris Ford

ISBN: 978-0-9568176-6-2
Published: Apr 2012, 268pp

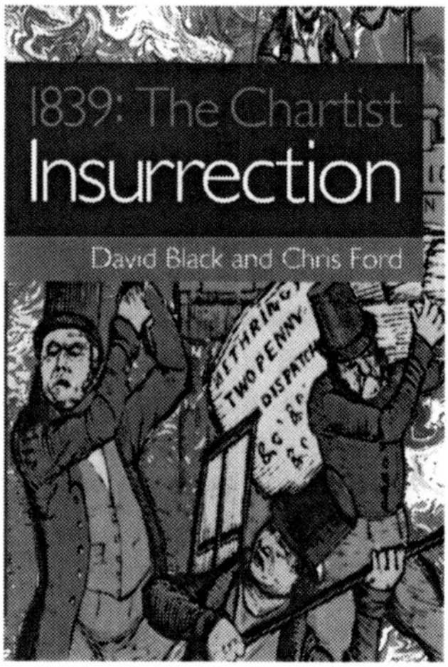

"With its meticulous attention to detailed sources, its comprehensive scope and its exacting research, this book doesn't just address the neglect of this important and interesting episode in Labour movement history, but more importantly it also challenges us to think again about the revolutionary potential of the British Labour movement."

John McDonnell MP, *Foreword*

In retrieving the suppressed history of the Chartist insurrection, David Black and Chris Ford have written a revolutionary handbook. Without romanticism or condescension, they track the difficulties of unifying local revolts without selling out to the 'representative politics' favoured in the parliamentary charade. As today's anti-capitalism faces the problem of anger without organisation, the lessons of the Chartists become crucial. Dialectics is not something to be derived from pure philosophy: by looking at the political problems of an insurgent working class, Black and Ford resurrect the true One-to-Many dialectic.

Association of Musical Marxists

The Struggle for Hearts and Minds: Essays on the Second World War

Ray Challinor

ISBN: 978-0-9568176-1-7
Published: Sep 2011, 128pp

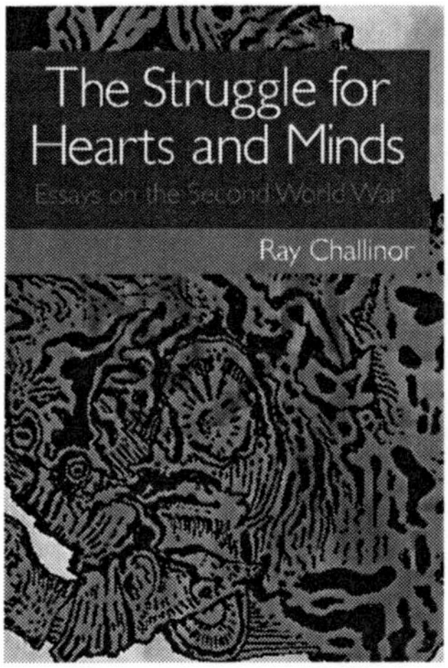

This book of essays is a shocking read, but the shocks arrive from the history itself, not sensationalist writing. We've been told that the Second World War was a war against evil waged by the goodhearted and true. The spectre of Hitler and Nazism is invoked every time NATO bombs are aimed at a defenceless country.

In his scathing account of ruling-class fears, plans and allegiances, Ray Challinor shows how much their every move was governed by competition and self-interest – and anxieties about popular reaction. His evidence shatters the comforting national myth which has been spun around the cataclysm – and shows that people, working-class people, do not like killing each other, they had to be cajoled and manipulated into doing so.

"*Read Ray Challinor's,* The Struggle for Hearts and Minds, *to learn the truth, not just about the Second World War, but of the eternal truth about war: They were bombing Iraqi villages in 1923.*"

Sharon Borthwick, *Unkant*

Happiness: Poems After Rimbaud

Sean Bonney

ISBN: 978-0-9568176-6-2
Published: Sep 2011, 128pp

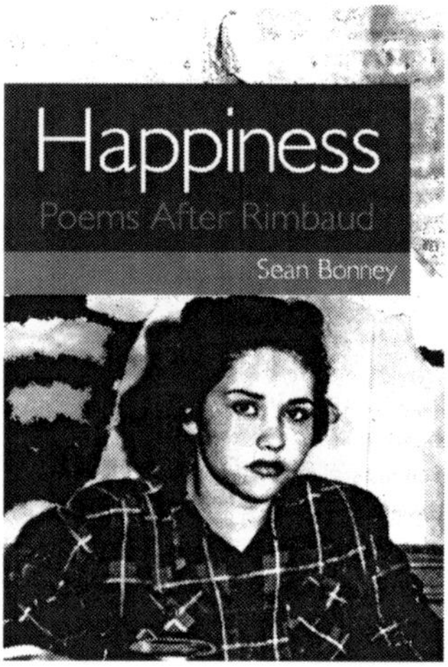

It is impossible to fully grasp Rimbaud's work, and especially *Une Saison en Enfer*, if you have not studied through and understood the whole of Marx's *Capital*. And this is why no English speaking poet has ever understood Rimbaud. Poetry is stupid, but then again, stupidity is not the absence of intellectual ability but rather the scar of its mutilation.

Rimbaud hammered out his poetic programme in 1871, just as the Paris Commune was being blown off the map. He wanted to be there. It's all he talked about. The *"systematic derangement of the senses"* is the social senses, ok, and the *"I"* becomes an *"other"* as in the transformation of the individual into the collective when it all kicks off. It's only in the English speaking world you have to point simple shit like that out. But then again, these poems have **NOTHING TO DO WITH RIMBAUD**. If you think they're translations you're an idiot. In the enemy language it is necessary to lie.

Adorno for Revolutionaries

Ben Watson

ISBN: 978-0-9568176-0-0
Published: May 2011, 256pp

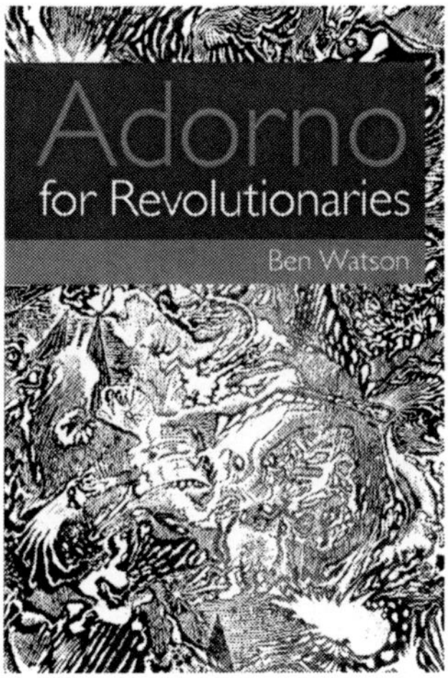

Starting with the commodity form (rather than the 'spirit' lauded by everyone from Classic FM retards to NME journalists), Adorno outlined a revolutionary musicology, a passageway between subjective feeling and objective conditions. In *Adorno for Revolutionaries,* Ben Watson argues that this is what everyone's been looking for since the PCF blackened the name of Marxism by wrecking the hopes of May '68. Batting aside postmodern prattlers and candyass pundits alike, this collection detonates the explosive core of Adorno's thought.

The **Association of Musical Marxists** says: Those 'socialists' who are frightened of their feelings can go stew in their imaginary bookshop. For us, great music is a necessity. To talk about it is to criticise everything that exists.

"*For those who have the ears to hear I strongly recommend* Adorno For Revolutionaries *as a substantial and very readable effort.*"

Dave Black, *Hobgoblin*

Lightning Source UK Ltd.
Milton Keynes UK
UKOW02f2357091216
289573UK00001B/8/P

9 780992 650902